Clinical
Leadership

ABOUT THE AUTHOR

Dickon Weir-Hughes joined the Nursing and Midwifery Council as Chief Executive and Registrar on 2 November 2009. Prior to this, he held a challenging turnaround appointment as Executive Director of Nursing/Professor of Nursing at Barking, Havering and Redbridge University Hospitals NHS Trust/London South Bank University.

Dickon is proud to have been Chief Nurse/Deputy Chief Executive at the world's leading cancer hospital, The Royal Marsden Hospital (London and Surrey), from 1998 to 2007, where he founded the Royal Marsden School of Nursing and Rehabilitation. He was responsible for clinical governance, patient safety and ICT, ran the UK National Cancer Leadership Programme and led on leadership development for nurses and midwives in the 97 trusts in London as the 'leading light' for the London SHA.

From 1994 to 1998 Dickon was Deputy Director of Nursing at Chelsea and Westminster Hospital, London. Prior to this, he had a varied clinical career at St. Bartholomew's Hospital, London and St. George's/ Atkinson Morley's Hospital, London. He was also a flight nurse for Europ Assistance and was one of the six nurses who went to Baghdad to repatriate sick and injured hostages at the start of the first Gulf War.

He is the elected President of NANDA International until 2012 (formerly the North American Nursing Diagnosis Association), a Non-Executive Director of the National Patient Safety Agency and the Chairman of the Foundation of Nursing Studies.

Clinical Leadership

from A to Z

Dickon Weir-Hughes

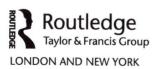

Routledge
Taylor & Francis Group

LONDON AND NEW YORK

First published 2011 by Pearson Education Limited

Published 2013 by Routledge
2 Park Square, Milton Park, Abingdon, Oxon OX14 4RN
711 Third Avenue, New York, NY 10017, USA

Routledge is an imprint of the Taylor & Francis Group, an informa business

ISBN 13: 978-0-273-75156-4 (pbk)

British Library Cataloguing-in-Publication Data
A catalogue record for this book is available from the British Library

Library of Congress Cataloging-in-Publication Data
A catalog record for this book is available from the Library of Congress

Typeset in 7.5pt Melior by 3

Contents

Introduction

Clinical leadership has always been challenging. Traditionally, healthcare has lacked the incentive structures of 'big business'; it is highly regulated and has suffered from overly rigid and sometimes illogical professional boundaries. In more recent times, the global financial climate, demographic and epidemiological developments, emerging technologies and managing an aging population have all provided additional challenges for healthcare leaders. However, within this perhaps bleak and unforgiving environment there are fantastic, exciting and rewarding leadership opportunities.

In this book I have used my personal experience of the 'sharp end' of clinical leadership in a number of organisations, all challenging in their own way, rather than taken a purely academic perspective. *Clinical Leadership* also draws on my experience as a leadership programme facilitator, mentor and coach. A frequently occurring theme from the participants of such programmes and others that I have had the privilege of working with is the need to grasp leadership concepts and terminology, to assess one's competence against such a framework and to have some suggestions for taking forward personal development. I have tried to provide a succinct summary of some of the key concepts of leadership in an accessible and manageable format together with some inspiration! The A to Z is designed to be a useful source of information for individuals on 360-degree leadership evaluation appraisals, leadership courses and modules and indeed for anyone faced with the challenge of clinical leadership and in need of a 'dip in and out of' resource.

Clinicians* have an opportunity, from early in their careers, to make an extraordinary difference to their patients. However, the decision to become a clinical leader is often born out of a strongly held desire to make a much greater difference to a greater number of patients, their loved ones, staff and students. Clinical leaders have the opportunity to set the tone of an organisation and to develop an environment where high-quality care can flourish. Having such an opportunity is a great honour.

Optimal leadership development is a never-ending, reflective journey. I hope that this resource aids you on *your* exciting journey as a clinical leader.

Professor Dickon Weir-Hughes
London, February 2011

* Throughout this book the term clinician is used to describe clinicians from all disciplines including, but not limited to, medical doctors, nurses, midwives, allied health professionals and pharmacists.

How to use this book

My driver for writing this book was to provide a helpful and practical summary of key leadership principles within healthcare. Its purpose is to be practical and accessible, so please feel free to use it as such! Use it as a resource book, scribble all over it, highlight sections, fold down corners, run reflective diaries alongside it.

Some suggested guidelines are:

- Dedicate a notebook to this book, and use it to jot down ideas, undertake the suggested exercises, and write notes from the suggested reading.

- Understand what it means to use/keep a reflective diary (Google it!), and then use a reflective diary as you read this book.

- Regardless of your professional background, use *International Textbook on Reflective Practice in Nursing*, Freshwater, D., Taylor, J. and Sherwood, G., Wiley-Blackwell, Oxford, 2008. Of particular interest should be Chapter 7, 'Reflective practice: the route to nursing leadership'.

Acknowledgements

My thanks go to the many healthcare professionals I have had the privilege to lead, manage and teach. You have taught me more than I could have imagined. You have all generously endured my sometimes clumsy attempts to perfect my leadership skills, and I thank you for allowing me that opportunity.

My thanks, too, to the many wise and experienced leaders who have so generously supported and mentored me over the last 25 years.

And finally, to my ultimate rock, soul mate, supporter and voice of reason, Simon Kateley.

Publisher's acknowledgements

The publisher would like to thank the following for their kind permission to reproduce their photographs:

Fotolia.com
Page 10 © Pix by Marti; Page 16 © gunnar3000; Page 24 © Marc Dietrich; Page 30 © Andres Rodriguez; Page 36 © SVLuma; Page 44 © Marek; Page 56 © Monkey Business; Page 62 © Irena Misevic; Page 68 © Stephen Coburn; Page 76 © deanm1974; Page 84 © nyul; Page 92 © Yuri Arcurs; Page 98 © S. Rae; Page 104 © Sean Gladwell; Page 124 © Chad McDermott; Page 136 © apops; Page 144 © Robert Mizerek; Page 158 © Maridav; Page 164 © Willee Cole; Page 170 © GIS.

Shutterstock.com
Page 2 © RTImages; Page 50 © Yuri Arcurs; Page 110 ©
Gunnar Pippel; Page 116 © iofoto; Page 130 © marekuliasz;
Page 150 © Pixsooz.

Every effort has been made to trace the copyright holders
and we apologise in advance for any unintentional
omissions. We would be pleased to insert the appropriate
acknowledgement in any subsequent edition of this
publication.

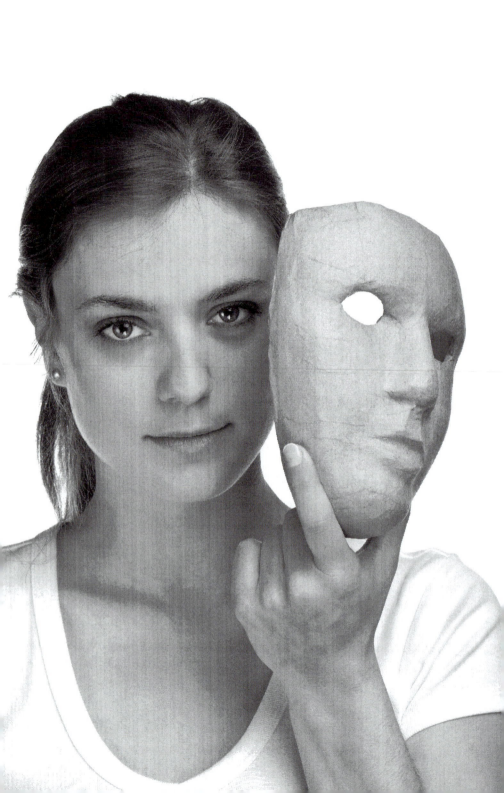

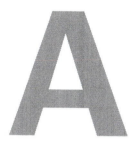

Authenticity

Be a first rate version of yourself, not a second rate version of someone else.

Judy Garland

Have you ever taken time to think about what leadership means, or what leadership *really* is? In their pursuit to answer this very question, Irvine and Reger interviewed many influential leaders, including clinicians, teachers, entrepreneurs and CEOs of multi-million pound businesses. They found the answer to their question ... and to ours. Leadership is not just about a job title, a particular position within an organisation, an individual's list of responsibilities or even their achievements. Great leadership is about 'inspiring, guiding and supporting others to be true to their own identity. It is about having a commitment and a capacity to encourage, support and guide other people through the strength of who *they* are.'[1] Frank Rich, in his study on Western society after the events of September 11, 2001, supported this definition by suggesting that 'people seek leaders who can restore confidence in basic institutions and enhance their confidence that they can collectively achieve a better, more secure world'.[2]

Ultimately, leadership is about providing the best environment in which the people you lead can flourish and grow. A great analogy of successful leadership can be found

1 Irvine, D. and Reger, J. *The Authentic Leader*, DC Press, Sanford, FL, 2006, p2.
2 Eagly, A.H. 'Achieving Relational Authenticity in Leadership: Does Gender Matter?', *Leadership Quarterly*, 2005, 16, pp459–474.

in gardening. No plant ever grew faster, taller or stronger just because the gardener demanded that it did so, or threatened it. Plants will only ever grow when the conditions are right and they receive the care they need to flourish. And the same is true with people. Creating the best environment for plants and for people requires providing continued attention and investment.[3] Individuals who provide that attention and investment can grow great leaders ... and great gardeners! Indeed, the key to effective leadership in healthcare is not just crafting an environment where people can thrive and grow, but essentially one which is therapeutic and where excellence in clinical care is a top priority.

However worthy, it can be difficult to put this definition of leadership into practice, especially when you need to establish yourself as a leader within an environment where the constant pressures of budgets, targets and local initiatives can mean that it's easier to be a dictatorial manager than a great leader. To support and inspire others to be true to their own values and beliefs, regardless of the external pressures they face on a day-to-day basis, means first leading by example. You need to be 'real', you need to be authentic. And you need to commit yourself to being grounded in reality, as opposed to acting on perception. The definition of behaving in an authentic way is to be trustworthy and reliable and to act independently. Being 'real' is about routinely exuding these qualities, and 'understanding [that] authenticity may help to identify outstanding leaders and to foster effective leadership through the design of appropriate training experiences'.[4]

Being true to yourself and your values will lead to trust and respect – both from yourself and from those you work with. Engaging with your colleagues in a way that demonstrates

3 See note 1, p64.
4 See note 2.

that your peers have your absolute attention, that you are
listening to them and that you are acting in a way that is
based on reality and therefore not based on a provided
perception, is inextricably linked to clinical competency and
is a fundamental part of behaving authentically. Interestingly
this is often described as 'presence' in the moment, and is a
skill that most clinicians possess and are able to demonstrate
beautifully. Think about instances in the past when you
have dealt with patients or carers. Patients and carers can
immediately tell if the clinician they are with is not really
'present' (in the moment), if they are not giving them their
full attention. It is vital to a patient's well-being and to
developing a therapeutic relationship that they feel heard
and that they have your undivided attention. Conveying
presence is an everyday skill that clinicians possess, and
one that is also crucial to successful leadership. It is a skill
that is critical to relieving and resolving the anxiety of
others and in effectively engaging with staff and undertaking
performance management. Presence engenders trust,
respect and commitment, and it forms an essential part of
authenticity. Being true to yourself, displaying the 'real you'
100 per cent of the time, enables you to encourage the same
level of honesty in your staff and peers.

Everyone has beliefs and values, characteristics and
viewpoints that make up their authentic self. They make
you who you are; ultimately they define you. And as Ken
Blanchard states, 'your beliefs are where you find the
essence of your leadership point of view. These should flow
naturally from the people who have influenced you, and
from your purpose and values.'[5] Becoming a leader does not
mean losing your values or suppressing your beliefs – indeed
it is the very opposite! It should mean leading through these
values, and encouraging others to do the same. Of course this

5 Blanchard, K. *Leading at a Higher Level*, FT Prentice Hall, Pearson, Harlow,
2007, p281.

can sound easy in principle and be a nightmare in practice. Moving from a clinical role to a leadership role is daunting, and a period of transition is to be expected and should be supported by your peers through personal and professional development, coaching and/or mentoring, and your own managerial support. Professional organisations also offer a range of support and development opportunities.

It can seem very easy to act a part when taking on a new role, especially a leadership role, and interestingly Eagly's study into authenticity suggests that, 'in many contexts, female leaders, more than male leaders, face challenges in achieving legitimacy as spokespersons for values that advance a community's interests'.[6] Similarly, leaders defined as 'outsiders', that is, groups of people or minority groups who have not traditionally had access to leadership roles, also find achieving an authentic leadership style difficult. The primary reason cited for this is a lack of belief on the part of the 'followers' that the leader's authentic self, values and views are right for the organisation. It can sometimes be difficult for women or minority group leaders to 'garner support for their agenda if they are not perceived as appropriate spokespersons for the community'.[7] Often this difficulty may not be 'real', but a difficulty that is perceived by the leader.

But it is very obvious to people if you are not authentic, and it can be negative and detrimental – to yourself, to those that you are there to support, and ultimately to patients and carers. Failing to lead through your values or adopting a fake exterior in the workplace can lead to losing sight of your core values and beliefs, and losing or never gaining trust from your peers and staff. Ultimately your leadership style

---

6 Eagly, A.H. 'Achieving Relational Authenticity in Leadership: Does Gender Matter?', *Leadership Quarterly*, 2005, 16, pp459–474.
7 See note above.

shifts from that of an effective leader to an implementer of management policy.

So, having grasped the importance of remaining authentic or 'being yourself' when leading others, the next step is to understand how to recognise when you are leading authentically. Irvine and Reger state that there are eight key qualities to authenticity, and whilst this is by no means an exhaustive list, it does at least provide a starting point on which you can build. Their eight key qualities of authenticity are:

Quality	Explanation
Clarity	Understanding the importance and power of focus Striving to find your own voice and purpose, and then encouraging others to do the same Keeping focused on the important things
Courage	Remaining true to yourself when those around you choose to 'put on an act' Trusting yourself and your direction
Integrity	Honestly, self-honesty and being accountable for your own actions
Service	Giving to others Understanding and the power of servant leadership
Trust	Trusting yourself and understanding how this affects self-confidence Understanding the importance of gaining the trust of others
Humility	Having an honest identity Practising modesty and realising that those with humility tend to have a strong inner confidence that is compelling and powerful

Quality	Explanation
Compassion	Caring for others and reaching out to others
Vulnerability	Being human Connecting with others on a human level Recognising and openly accepting that you make mistakes and that you will face uncertainties throughout your life

Source: Data from Irvine, D. and Reger, J. *The Authentic Leader*, DC Press, Sanford, FL, 2006, pp109–168.

Taking authenticity forward

▎ Use the table above to think about your leadership style. How do you work with and develop your staff? How do you lead your team? Are you grounded in the present when you're leading your team? Are you true to your values and beliefs and do you encourage others to do the same? Do you lead authentically?

▎ Study one of the texts suggested in this chapter.

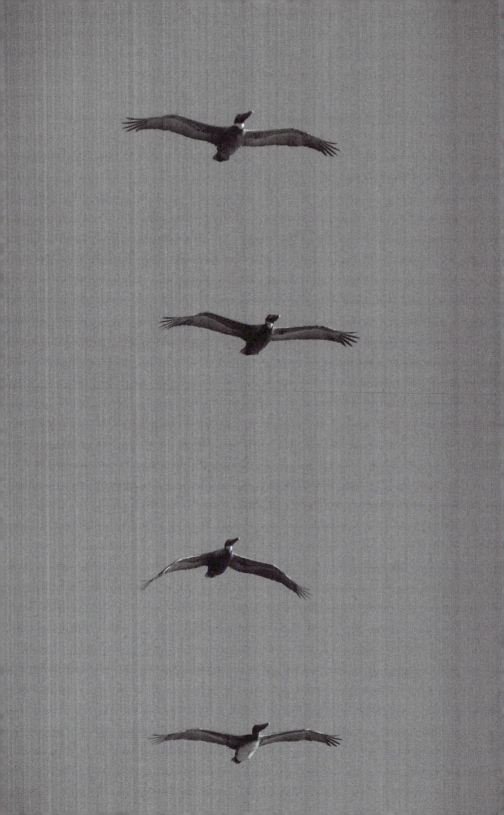

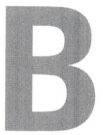

Behaviour

Ability may get you to the top, but it takes character to keep you there.

John Wooden

A person's behaviour is the principal factor that determines how others perceive them. Behaviour is characteristically an external demonstration of a person's core values and beliefs. However, behaviour can be moderated to enable an individual to adapt to a situation or environment or, indeed, so that they are perceived by others in a different light. Good leaders are often followed because they are deemed to be trustworthy and committed to their cause. However, this is often a judgement based on the leader's behaviour and not necessarily their skills. Leadership is primarily about behaviour first and skills second. It sounds clichéd but a successful leader should behave in line with the sentiment that they treat others as they would expect to be treated.

In order that an individual can behave as a good leader, they have to possess a full and conscious understanding of their own values and beliefs. Self-awareness will help you as a leader to understand and analyse your own leadership experiences and so enhance your maturity and wisdom. This understanding will also allow you to develop your personal leadership skills for the future. Clarifying your own beliefs is also a crucial part of the leadership development journey. Whilst your skills may change over time, your core values and beliefs, such as the primacy of caring for others, will probably remain constant. Holding onto your core values and beliefs, whilst respecting those of others, is vital to allow you to adapt to and overcome the leadership challenges that you will face.

Understanding your own values is obviously extremely important but it is also vital you are open to understanding other people's values. This therefore implies that an effective leader should be interested in the people they are leading. This interest must be deep and genuine, in order that you can understand, coach and develop people to achieve their maximum potential within your organisation. Individual values and experiences will all add to the diversity and the richness that a workforce can bring to an organisation and you should therefore welcome the wide array of beliefs and viewpoints that occur within the workplace. Everyone can benefit from others' knowledge and life experiences and they can help you to not only enhance the team you are leading but also enable you to become a better leader. However, an important part of the leader's role is to bring some of these possibly disparate views together to enable the group to deliver their service.

The first steps to understanding and learning about others and their values is to learn to listen effectively. 'If you are seen to be hearing rather than listening then people will ask themselves not only whether you have really heard what is being said but also if you have sufficient commitment to the change.'[8] In essence then, if you do not behave in a genuine manner, expressing a real interest in others' thoughts and opinions, then those that you are leading will doubt your ability to carry out the tasks that they are asking of you. Alongside active listening there should also be frequent and honest communication. It is good practice not only to offer

---

8 Goodwin, N. *Leadership in Health Care: A European Perspective*, Routledge Health Management Series, Routledge, London and New York, 2006, p171.

feedback to your colleagues but also to ask them for honest feedback on your leadership skills and, importantly, for you to act upon the advice given; in some circumstances this may result in you having to change your behaviour.

In addition to changing your behaviour as a result of feedback received from colleagues, you should also personally assess whether any of your leadership behaviours should or could be moderated. Moderation in this context means developing your skills in one leadership behaviour in order to positively change a leadership behaviour that presents a challenge. A 360-degree evaluation, such as the LEA (Leadership Effectiveness Analysis tool),[9] can often help to determine which leadership behaviours require development. For example, becoming expert at appropriate delegation can result in a leader being less controlling and thus positively changing their behaviour.

Once you have understood your core beliefs and communicated with those you are leading it is vital to make sure that you are a visible role model to others. Visibility and 'walking the talk' is key to the role of an effective leader. An effective leader should consider their 'constituents' – the people who impact on their role or who they need to network with to make their role a success. It is important to be clear about who your constituents are as a leader, recognising that your most important constituents may be outside the organisation. Your constituents will consist of a range of individuals, some more senior to you in the hierarchy and others 'junior' to you; but all will possess a unique set of core values and life experiences. You should make a calculated decision to make yourself visible to your constituents and allocate time to spend with colleagues so that you are able to reflect your own values and behaviour on others around you.

9 www.mrg.com/products/leadership.asp, Management Research Group.

With this visibility as a leader you will constantly be on show and, as such, you should be aware of the way in which your genuine personality blends with the role you play when you are 'acting the part' of leader. For any leader to work effectively, your constituents need to predominantly see your true personality. Different roles, organisations and situations will require you to sometimes adapt your behaviour but you should always work to the values of authenticity, honesty, openness and integrity. If you can behave in such a way that you are being true to yourself but also being seen as an effective leader by others, then you will possess the behavioural tools necessary to succeed.

Taking behaviour forward

▌ Influence your line manager to allow you to participate in a 360-degree evaluative process and develop a personal development action plan for yourself based on the results.

▌ Reflect on the behaviour of a leader for whom you have great respect. What is it about them that makes them such a great leader?

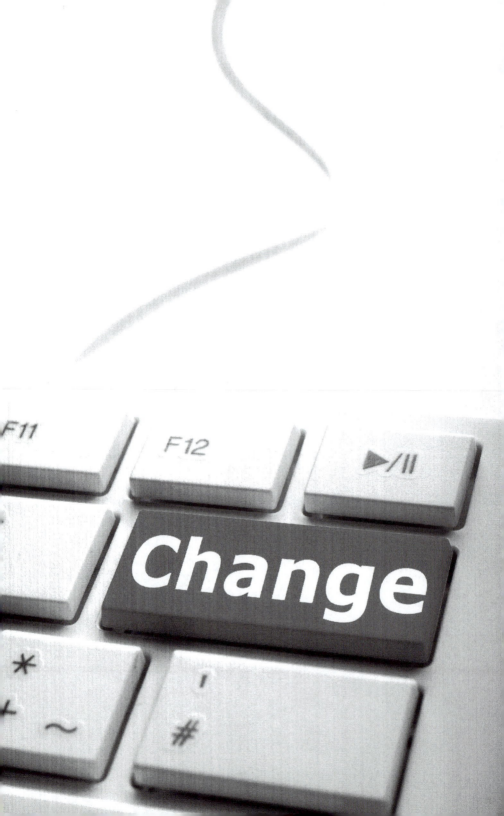

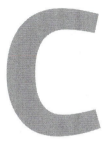

Change management

The main dangers in this life are the people who want to change everything or nothing.

Lady Nancy Astor

n order to understand how to manage change effectively we must first consider how and when change occurs. 'Change can be defined as making the form, nature, or content etc of something different from what it is or from what it would be if left alone.'[10] This definition can be applied to a vast array of situations that may arise within a healthcare setting, from a change in staffing structure to a change in best practice guidelines. Change can be significant and affect the masses or it can be small and its impact may be considered negligible by the majority. Managing any change effectively regardless of its scale involves the use of well thought out processes and the careful implementation of a structured plan. The implications and the process of change should be considered in its entirety to ensure that all potential negative impacts of the change have been assessed and minimised as far as possible. To carry out such an assessment and then monitor the outcome of the change requires some quantitative or qualitative scale to be in place. 'Change must be realistic, achievable and measurable.'[11]

The idea that change requires effective management primarily originates from the work of Everett Rogers who developed

10 www.dictionary.reference.com
11 www.businessballs.com/changemanagement.htm

a theory within his book, *Diffusion of Innovations.*[12] Rogers considered there to be five stages, which an innovation or change goes through, from its initial conception to its implementation. He has redefined the terms used to describe these stages over the years, and they are now referred to as follows:

1. **Knowledge** – the idea that there is potential for innovation is acknowledged but there is a specific lack of information to allow this to occur.

2. **Persuasion** – the innovation is developed at this stage through an individual actively seeking further information, which allows them to progress intelligently to stage 3.

3. **Decision** – the advantages and disadvantages of implementing the innovation are considered and a decision is then made as to whether to proceed.

4. **Implementation** – the innovation or change is made and its effect in terms of its positive and negative outcomes is then assessed.

5. **Confirmation** – the decision is then finalised and at this time the innovation can be used to its fullest potential.

This five-stage process clearly describes a well planned and executed change. To allow change to occur whilst ignoring such a process can be extremely detrimental to your organisation and to your credibility as a leader. Failing to manage change may result in the change not yielding the desired outcome and consequently staff and patients may feel that the change has not improved their experience or healthcare delivery in any way. This could cause bad feeling amongst them, which will ultimately be directed towards the leader initiating the change.

---

12 Rogers, E.M. *Diffusion of Innovations*, 4th edition, Free Press, New York, 2003.

Change will inevitably occur at many levels, from government-led changes affecting the whole of society, to organisation-wide changes, through to changes within your department or team. It is important to understand that change will always be necessary to ensure that healthcare and professionals remain forward-thinking and proactive in providing the best possible service to patients. However, human nature makes many people cautious about change and many will be reluctant or averse to adopting change. 'We live in a society that seems to resist change. Even though we're surrounded by tens of millions of other species that demonstrate wonderful capacities to grow, adapt, and change.'[13] Learning to adapt to change is an important behaviour for everyone working in healthcare. Therefore, as a leader, you must be able to implement and manage change effectively so that those people who are cautious or change-averse can feel comfortable and secure with the changes made. Without a calculated and measured process in place, your staff may react negatively to the positive changes you are attempting to introduce. There is the risk that those you are leading will simply ignore your changes or actively oppose them. An effective leader needs to apply appropriate strategies and behaviour to address individuals' concerns or issues around the change. Frequently these issues have arisen through a lack of knowledge surrounding the reasons for the change and the expected and desired outcomes. Referring back to Rogers' model, it could be considered wise to allow those who will be impacted by the change to be a part of the five-stage process.

There are many varying techniques written about change management, all of which aim to minimise the disruption that can be caused by change and allow for its positive acceptance.

13 Wheatley, M.J. *Leadership and the New Science: Discovering Order in a Chaotic World*, 2nd edition, Berrett-Koehler, San Francisco, 1999, p138.

Many organisations have change management incorporated into their policies. This will be a tried and tested means of managing change effectively and should therefore be adhered to at all times. One change management technique that provides a comprehensive way of dealing with change can be seen in the theory of 'Directional Leadership – Recommended Action'. This technique highlights the importance of first ensuring that the whole leadership team is engaged with the change. It suggests that people react to change in a manner that mirrors how their leaders react; therefore if some leaders are not in total support of the change this could cause followers to react in a similar fashion. It is vital that the leadership team 'thrash out' their differences in private and then present a united front. Secondly, this technique recommends that as a leader you should ensure that everyone is aware of the reason for the change. Individuals do not have to agree with the change but if they are aware of the reasons behind it, this will facilitate its acceptance. In the same way, if they are aware of how the change will directly impact on them as individuals then, again, they will be more willing to embrace it. The final recommendation of this technique is to introduce change as an improvement rather than a change; this simple adjustment in terminology can often help employees to see the effects of change in a more beneficial light.

Seeing through and delivering change requires a leader to be clear and confident. To effectively manage change and to engage those that it affects requires a leader to adopt a proven technique, which allows for careful consideration and controlled implementation. The leader must themselves be knowledgeable and enthusiastic about the change and its benefits in order that they can inspire others to react in a similar vein.

Taking change management forward

▌ Consider and reflect upon a change you have been subjected to and that you didn't support. How did this make you feel as a recipient of change?

▌ Consider and reflect upon a change you have initiated, and been responsible for implementing (it doesn't matter how minor the change was). How did you feel and what would you have done differently or better?

▌ Gain a thorough understanding of your organisation's policies on change management.

▌ Study one of the texts referred to in this chapter.

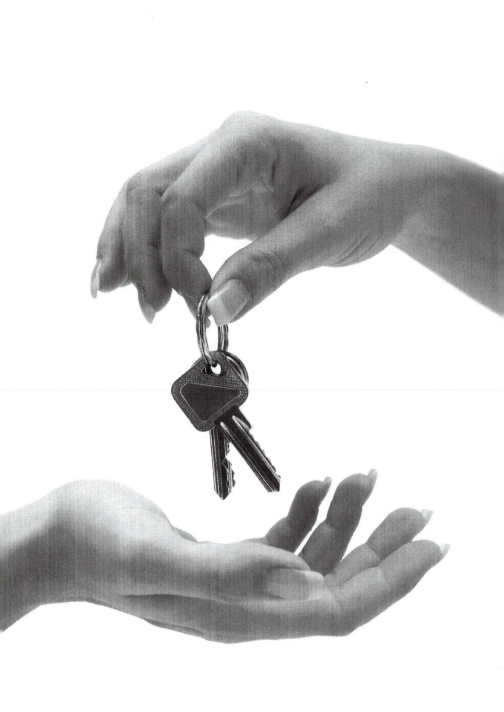

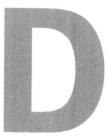

Delegation

The best executive is the one who has sense enough to pick good men to do what he wants done, and self-restraint enough to keep from meddling with them while they do it.

Theodore Roosevelt

Delegation is the means by which a leader can share out or transfer responsibilities to others. There are many reasons why a leader should delegate and, if dealt with properly, delegation can have many benefits for the delegator, the person delegated to and the leader's team as a whole. One of the more common reasons why a leader will delegate is because they are overwhelmed with the quantity of their work or because they are aware that with their current workload they will be unable to meet a specific deadline. This reason, although a valid one, could highlight possible failures within leadership technique; workloads should be planned and resourced appropriately from the outset and although sometimes it is unavoidable, a leader should make every effort not to reach the situation where they are overwhelmed. Another reason for delegation is to stretch and develop members of your team. Offering staff the opportunity to undertake tasks delegated to them creates good working relationships as they are made aware that they are trusted with greater responsibility. Being awarded this trust often results in the staff member applying extra effort to fulfil the delegated task successfully. To achieve this success the staff member develops their own personal skills, expertise and confidence in their abilities, which in turn benefits the team and the organisation as a whole. Through such delegation individuals can learn to become

leaders and you can plan for this shift from follower to
leader gradually by assessing individuals' strengths as they
complete delegated tasks. A further benefit of delegation
is that leaders can be unburdened from mundane, routine
tasks, which allows for more time to be allocated to more
important leadership tasks that cannot always be delegated.
This type of delegation practice makes for effective time
management too!

Most leaders with clinical backgrounds are well accustomed
to delegating in clinical areas but there are a number
of considerations to be managed if one is to perfect
delegation skills. It is important for a leader to be aware
that not all tasks are always suitable for delegation – for
example, serious conflict management. It is also important
for a leader to make the correct choice with regard to
who they delegate tasks to. The appropriate allocation of
tasks requires a sound knowledge of your team's skills
and experiences. Delegating tasks inappropriately may
have a detrimental effect; for example, the task may not
be completed effectively and will therefore have to be
reassigned or passed back to you as a leader to resolve.
There is also the negative impact on the person delegated
to, as they become conscious of the fact that they have
failed at the task entrusted to them, which will knock
their confidence in their abilities. They may also feel
that this failure is the fault of their leader due to the
inadequate provision of guidance or support. To delegate
effectively, therefore, a leader must choose an individual
who possesses suitable skills, experience and motivation to
complete the task. The task must then be explained fully,
including a discussion about any background information
concerning the reasons for delegation and the importance of
the task at large, so that it can be seen in context. Finally,
'throughout the time that the person is undertaking the task,
you [their leader] should be available to give the person

advice, support and guidance.'[14] This support is essential to enable the process of delegation to work effectively and for everyone involved to reap all of the potential benefits. 'Support don't abdicate – delegation doesn't mean that you withdraw completely from the task, instead you need to provide support and encouragement to the individual so that they are able to successfully complete the task.'[15]

An effective leader should also retain some control throughout the task to assess progress and to confirm that instructions have been fully understood and are being carried out in line with expectations. There are many guidelines concerning the best way for a leader to handle delegation but some key concepts include ensuring that it is dealt with positively and openly, and that all involved are aware of their expectations, and the provision of support and guidance throughout the completion of the delegated work piece or project.

Delegation is not, however, always an easy act to implement. 'Many clinical managers have difficulty delegating due to attitudes and values that they hold.'[16] Some leaders feel unable to relinquish complete control as they simply do not trust anyone else to be able to complete the task as well as they would. This is because they do not believe that anyone else has adequate expertise. This becomes demoralising for the team as they feel that their skills are not valued and it also makes the leader's workload potentially unmanageable; the leader again becomes overwhelmed with tasks that they should not be fulfilling, which distracts from the tasks that they should be completing. Another common cause of leaders failing to delegate is due to them feeling that in the time

14 Barker, A.M., Sullivan, D.T. and Emery, M.J. *Leadership Competencies for Clinical Managers: The Renaissance of Transformational Leadership*, Jones and Bartlett, London, 2005, p86.
15 www.teal.org.uk
16 See note 14, p85.

it takes them to explain the task required they could have completed it themselves. Although this may be true, a leader should always consider delegation within a wider spectrum and be aware that teaching an employee now could mean they are able to repeat the task independently in the future. Some leaders are also cautious of delegating because they do not wish to burden their team with extra responsibilities, particularly if they feel their department is already stretched. Within all of the above-mentioned situations, remember to take time to consider the positive outcomes of delegation, with regard to both your team and the service you are providing. Allowing a shift in responsibilities will result in you becoming a more effective leader. In addition, team morale can increase as trust and confidence grows, and ultimately there will be a subsequent improved service delivery.

The best delegators are probably those leaders who can balance delegation and control so as to allow their staff to develop new skills and take burdensome work forward, whilst retaining just enough control to ensure delivery. Sometimes this level of delegation and control has to be filtered in accordance with individual skills and experience, the importance of the task and the timeframe.

Taking delegation forward

▌ Having considered this chapter, self-assess your own delegation skills. Can you identify situations in which you could have done better? Can you identify situations in which you got the balance of delegation and control absolutely right? If so, what characterised that situation? How can you replicate it? You may wish to keep some reflective notes.

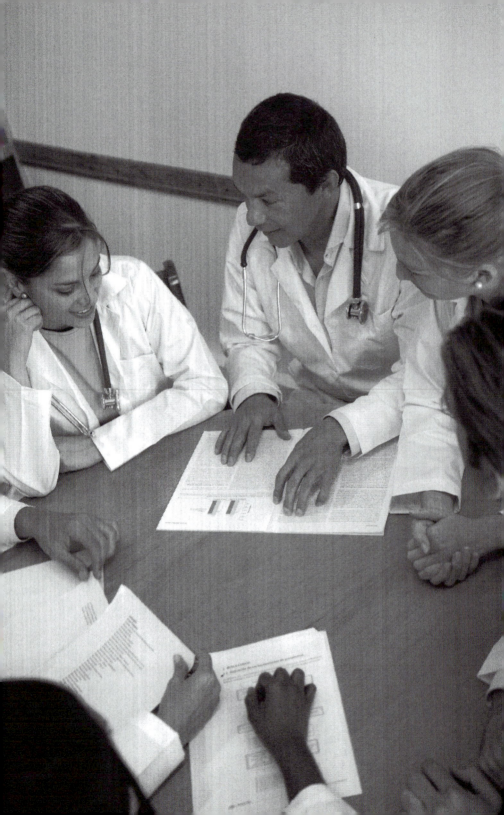

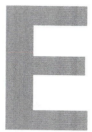

Engagement

Coming together is the beginning. Keeping together is progress. Working together is success.

Henry Ford

'The era of cascade, push, command and control is over. Employees need to be consulted, involved and inspired to live up to their potential.'[17] Engagement often provides that necessary sense of purpose which motivates individuals to apply themselves that little bit extra. For example, a member of domiciliary staff may work far more thoroughly if they are engaged and understand the impact that their work has on patient care and the successful running of the hospital as a whole. Engagement allows staff to understand exactly what they are working towards and how their efforts affect the organisation as a whole.

Sharing information and including staff in debates concerning change or working practices ensures that individuals are engaged with the whole business of healthcare and subsequently feel a sense of accountability for their work within the organisation. The importance of engagement within an organisation or a department should never be underestimated. Research has proven that there are many benefits to having an engaged workforce. These benefits include boosting morale within a team and improving individual levels of job satisfaction; this is due to the importance of each individual's input being acknowledged and everyone becoming aware of each other's significance within the team.

Engagement allows for lines of communication to be opened: this encourages feedback, which in turn helps organisations and leaders to develop and grow. In addition, it should also be recognised that the key to successful engagement *is* communication. 'Sharing information and facilitating open communication builds trust and encourages people to act like owners of the organisation.'[18] Having information readily available and encouraging open communication are the first steps towards achieving engagement. 'The more readily available information is, the more empowered and able people are to make solid decisions aligned with the organisation's goals and values.'[19]

Expert leaders are usually mindful of using their discretion regarding exactly how much information should be shared. An expert leader will be sufficiently politically aware of the impact of sharing certain information which, for example, may be of a sensitive nature. The aim should be to strive towards full engagement whenever possible but always remaining aware that sharing some details may not be appropriate.

In most situations engagement should be fully embraced and one of these situations is during times of change. Encouragement at the initial stages of the change will allow for alternative opinions and ideas to be presented and debated. 'If we fail to do this well, we not only risk disengaging our staff at this critical time, but will also miss out on benefiting from the intelligence that sits right across our organisation. Very often it's the person at the sharp end

---

18 Blanchard, K. *Leading at a Higher Level*, FT Prentice Hall, Pearson, Harlow, 2007, p10.
19 See note above.

who will have that brilliant idea that would really make a difference.'[20]

Having discussed the importance of engagement and the concept that communication is key to achieving it, the process by which a leader promotes this communication and facilitates engagement should now be considered. To achieve engagement takes time and effort and any leader looking to engage should make a conscious effort not only to talk to their staff but also to spend time understanding their roles and the individuals' skills. An effective leader should always ensure that they are readily available to their team to allow for two-way communication and feedback, which should not only be heard but also acted upon. Another essential point to recognise is that staff can only engage if they have the energy and enthusiasm to contribute that additional effort. In order to facilitate this, leaders should try to ensure that staff all have an acceptable work–life balance so that they are more capable of applying themselves in the workplace.

Once engagement is achieved the next step is to ensure that it is maintained. It can often seem easy to engage staff when there are significant changes ahead which will have a direct impact on them. However, to engage staff with respect to less significant day-to-day tasks can prove tricky and maintaining engagement year after year is an extremely difficult feat. As an individual's years of service increase, research has shown that the levels of engagement are certain to decrease. It is the leader's place therefore to act as the catalyst for maintaining constant engagement and also to monitor that it is actually occurring. Often leaders acknowledge that their staff have a significant influence over the development of their organisation but they do not proactively assess the actual contribution that their staff provide. As such, they

20 http://www.guardian.co.uk/values/socialaudit/story/0,,1932499,00.html#article_continue

are assuming that their staff are engaged and having their opinions heard, when in fact there is not a process in place for this to occur. It is the leader's responsibility therefore to make sure that there are processes in place to allow for effective engagement.

Leaders should consider engaging staff at every possible opportunity and should appreciate the contribution that their staff can make, accepting that the diversity within a workplace brings with it a wealth of opinions and viewpoints, which could provide a positive influence on your department, organisation and patients within your care.

Taking engagement forward

▎ Think about how you engage with patients, peers, staff and leaders. How could you improve these relationships to increase engagement levels?

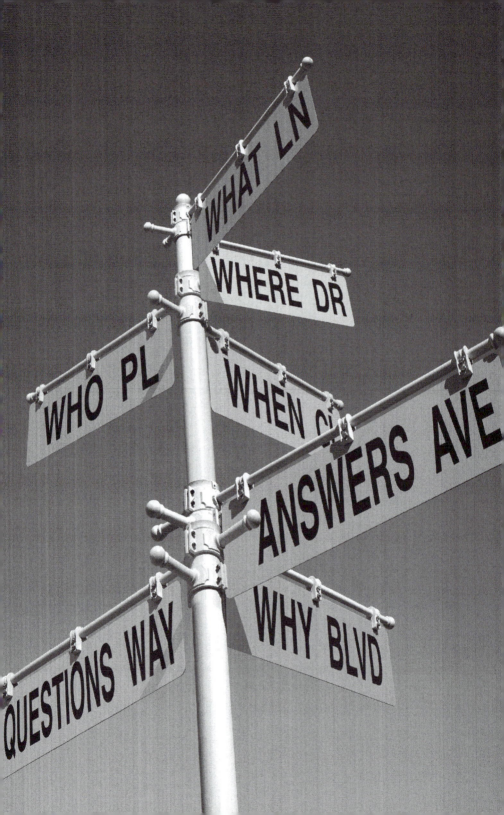

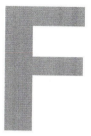

Feedback

Feedback is the breakfast of champions.

Ken Blanchard

Establishing a process for providing regular and constructive feedback is important for both staff and leaders. Feedback can be a means of praising good work and behaviour and there are many benefits of doing so. Providing positive feedback to staff boosts morale and also helps you as a leader define how you would like your team to work and the standards that you expect of them. Giving positive feedback is a relatively easy and enjoyable task, as it is welcomed by the individual receiving the feedback. Informing individuals of negative behaviours, however, can be more difficult and requires a somewhat different approach. Negative feedback which addresses ineffective or inappropriate behaviours, although it can be difficult to both give and receive, does serve a purpose. Informing individuals of negative feedback allows them the opportunity to take action to improve their working practices or behaviours, which will ultimately improve the service that they, their team and their organisation provides. Feedback has been defined as 'a way of helping another person change their behaviour'.[21]

It is important to acknowledge that as a leader there are some behaviours that *you* may need to change and you should therefore welcome feedback from your staff. For any leader, feedback should always be a two-way process – you both give and receive it. A good leader should encourage constructive feedback from their staff in order to improve their daily working life and also to assess how they are perceived as a leader. Feedback received from staff and given to a leader is known as upward feedback and is a recognised leadership practice: 'employees can provide useful input on the effectiveness of procedures and processes as well as input to managers on their leadership effectiveness'.[22]

When receiving feedback, the receiver should try to ensure that they handle the feedback with an open mind and should be prepared to change their behaviour if it is deemed necessary. When giving feedback it should always be in a constructive manner and it should be clear and specific and ultimately have a purpose, that is, to improve behaviours or indeed maintain good behaviours. To be given exact detail about where an individual is doing well or not so well is much more productive than giving vague, sweeping statements about an individual's behaviour. Always try to use practical examples that you have observed personally rather than general hearsay. There are occasions, however, when individuals are deprived from receiving important feedback, as it often makes people uncomfortable to comment on someone else's behaviour, particularly if it is negative. Usually individuals do not want to hurt the feelings of those they work with or for, as they anticipate that this will be harmful to their working relationships and team morale. However, to provide false feedback in order to save someone's feelings is a pointless activity and would ultimately be detrimental to your team, as ineffective behaviours will not be highlighted and will therefore remain. Individuals must therefore be guided in how to provide feedback in a productive manner. For example, if it is necessary to deliver negative feedback, you should try to balance this with a positive comment or spin in order that your feedback becomes motivating rather than demoralising. This is sometimes known as a 'praise sandwich', an example of which might be, 'You handled that meeting really well overall. It's important though to keep your cool with the Finance Director. Overall you were excellent though, thank you.'

Many staff will welcome feedback as they see it as an opportunity to gain valuable insight as to how they are performing and how they are perceived within their team. For most, feedback is a developmental process which allows individuals to measure how well their performance is matching expectations. There is, however, an argument against the merits of feedback due to the fact that it concentrates on events that have already occurred. Reflecting back in this way can be seen by some as very static and limiting. A way of combating this is to try 'feedforward'.[23] This practice involves choosing an area in which you as a leader or one of your staff wishes to improve. Then the various approaches and methods that could be used in order to achieve success in that area will be discussed as a group. Some individuals prefer taking a more proactive position such as this as they view it as being far more productive in being able to change the way they handle a future assignment rather than reflecting on how they handled a task in the past, which cannot be changed (although it could be argued that changes could be applied to the way they would handle the assignment in the future). In addition, feedforward is generally not taken as personally as feedback, as it is not direct comment on an individual's behaviour, more an open discussion about the ways in which an individual could behave, followed by a decision being made on the best approach. This therefore should not hurt anyone's feelings and will avoid the occurrence of false feedback.

The issues and difficulties around providing constructive feedback are encountered in all organisations and at all levels. 'Giving and receiving feedback are among the most complex and least understood leadership dilemmas confronting most managers today.'[24] Some of these perceived difficulties can be overcome through establishing a system of feedback within your team and highlighting the purpose of the feedback process. Informing staff of the reasons why feedback is invaluable and the fact that it needs to be regular and honest will be the first step towards encouraging constructive and meaningful feedback for both your staff and yourself as a leader.

There is one final area to consider in relation to receiving feedback, which links to a number of other leadership behaviours. Many healthcare professionals have been socialised by patients and families giving them frequent and positive feedback. As you become a more senior and established leader you will find that you do not get this level of positive feedback. Indeed, you may find that weeks slip by without anyone saying anything very nice to you at all! You will therefore need to develop as a more self-reliant and independent individual, throwing off any remnants of co-dependency and the need to be praised regularly.

Taking feedback forward

▌ Reflect on a situation in which you have provided feedback. How could you have been more effective? What was the outcome?

Reflect on a situation in which you know you have failed to provide the feedback you ought to have done, either to your boss or to a team member. Why didn't you feedback? What stopped you? Write a brief plan of how you intend to address this outstanding situation.

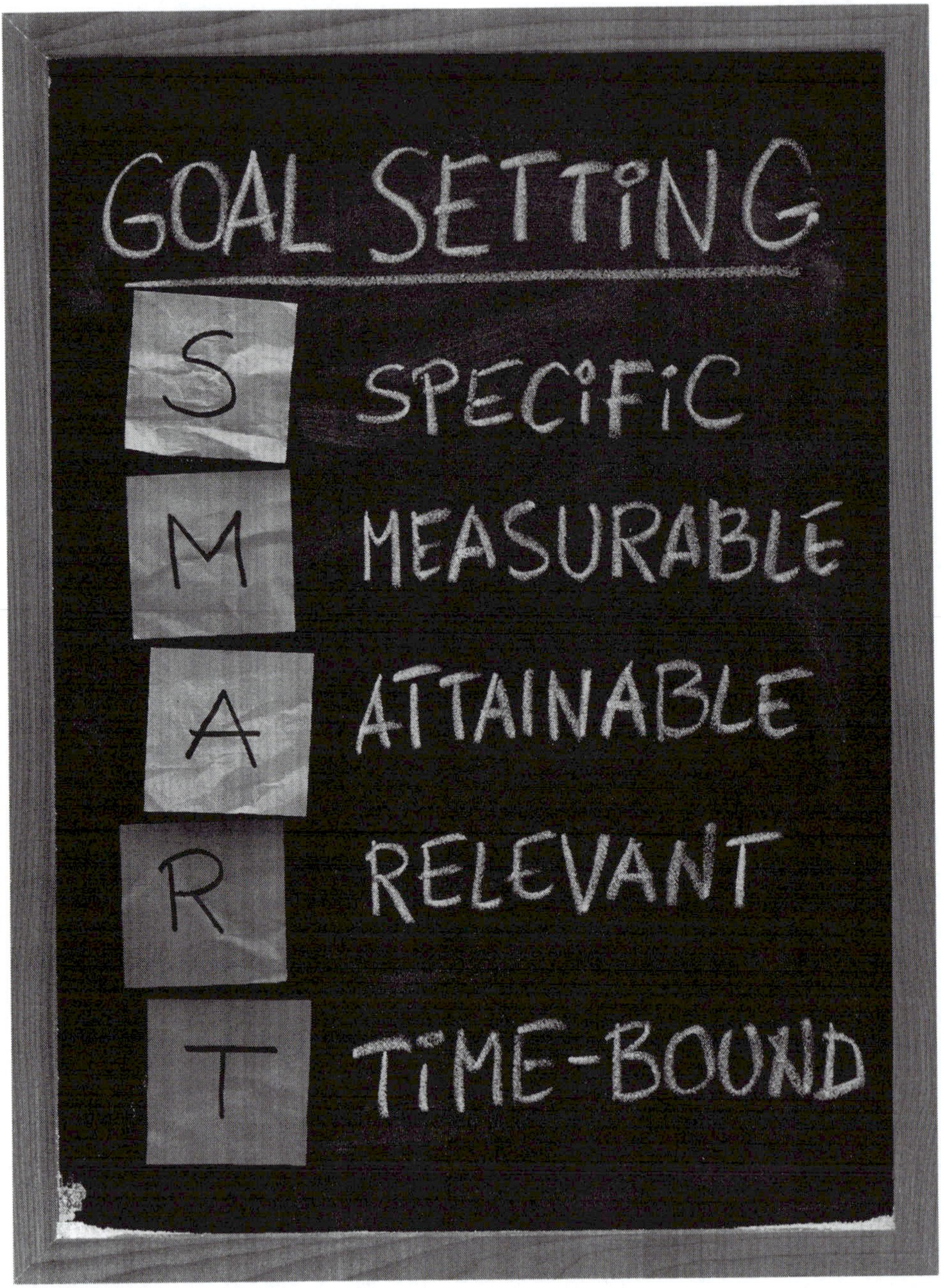
GOAL SETTING
S SPECIFIC
M MEASURABLE
A ATTAINABLE
R RELEVANT
T TIME-BOUND

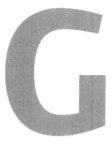

Goals

Become a possibilitarian. No matter how dark things seem to be or are, raise your sights and see possibilities – always see them, for they're always there.

Norman Vincent Peale

To have defined goals to work towards and achieve is essential both for yourself as a leader and for the team that you are leading. Goal setting, if done in the correct manner, provides a focus to your work, motivates individuals to achieve their goals, and allows for constant monitoring and a starting point around which you can initiate feedback. All of these direct consequences of working with goals results in a more effective service provision. There is a commonly used method that can be followed when setting goals to ensure that they are realistic and achievable. A commonly used acronym for the best way to set goals is SMART, which relates to the following terms.

- **Specific** – setting specific goals, that is, a goal that is not vague and open to misinterpretation, allows you to focus your mind on a structured task. It is vital to make sure that this specific goal is also measurable so that you have a clear point at which you can see that the goal has been achieved.

- **Measurable and motivating** – goals should push the boundaries of the achievements you easily make on a daily basis; they should be focused on tasks or standards you wish to achieve in order to improve yourself as a person or to improve the service you provide. A key to setting

goals that are motivating is to ultimately set goals that will
personally inspire you to want to achieve them.

▌ **Attainable** – whilst stretching boundaries it is imperative
that the goals should still be attainable. It is considered
detrimental to set goals that are unattainable as it then
becomes demoralising and individuals feel as though
they are underachieving even though they are delivering
their best. Therefore by not setting attainable goals you
will achieve the direct opposite of the outcomes you are
expecting.

▌ **Relevant** – goals should be relevant in terms of an
individual's personal and professional development and
with respect to the targets that your team are working
towards.

▌ **Time-bound** – this final point sets a limit on the time
within which it is expected that a goal should be achieved
and also allows for progress to be monitored as an
individual works towards their goal. Having a time-bound
goal or a deadline provides more focus and enhances an
individual's motivation.

It is important to set goals that inspire but you should ensure
that you limit the number of short-term goals that you set.
Having too many short-term goals can be detrimental, as the
desire to achieve goals could become the main focus of your
attention which could then distract from your other routine
duties or the unexpected tasks that come your way during
the course of your day. As a guide therefore it is advisable
to set three short-term goals that are a little stretch, in terms
of the effort required for you to achieve them, and then set
as many long-term goals as you want, ensuring of course
that these too are time-bound, even if they fall into a five- or
ten-year plan. Three to five goals are the ideal number on
which peak performers can concentrate, according to most

research.[25] Once you have set your goals you may wish to reveal them to others in your team. This makes the goals seem real and also adds towards motivating you to achieve them. In addition, if others are aware of your goals then they can also act to help you achieve them, resulting in the team working together towards achieving goals that are relevant and beneficial.

As a leader you will be responsible not only for helping members of your team to set their own goals but also for monitoring their progress towards achieving them. One means by which you can carry out both of these tasks is through regular, formal appraisal. Appraisals can be a good opportunity for review, development and communication. Within an appraisal, the 'appraisee' can identify how and where they have performed well or poorly in the previous period and can then go on to identify areas where they would like to improve in the future. The obvious next step then is for you as a leader to work with the 'appraisee' to set SMART goals in order that these improvements can be realised.

Another means by which you as a leader or your team members can agree and monitor personal and professional development goals is through the use of Personal Development Plans (PDPs). 'Personal Development Planning (PDP) is a structured process undertaken by an individual in the workplace to reflect upon their own learning, performance and to plan for their personal, educational and career development.'[26] The main objective for PDPs is to improve the capacity of individuals to understand their knowledge and career development in order that they can review, plan and take responsibility for their own learning.

25 Blanchard, K. *Leading at a Higher Level*, FT Prentice Hall, Pearson, Harlow, 2007, p149.
26 www.qualityresearchinternational.com

This review process incorporates the setting and monitoring of goals, which will in turn allow them to become more effective within the team.

As a leader you should encourage a formalised process of setting and monitoring goals. Goals should be set in line with the SMART process and should be monitored through regular feedback or other means such as appraisals; at all times the goals and the progress should be formally recorded. If the guidelines for the use of goals are adhered to, then the goals will work as useful tools in setting standards and motivating both yourself and your team.

Taking goals forward

▌ Review your own objectives. Do they adhere to SMART standards?

▌ Develop a private Personal Development Plan (in addition to one you may have at work) using SMART goals. You may not wish to share this with your manager but instead use it to guide your own development as a leader. Be really honest with yourself and review your progress regularly.

▌ Write your own retirement leaving speech. What do you hope to achieve in your career as a healthcare leader? What will people say of your achievements?

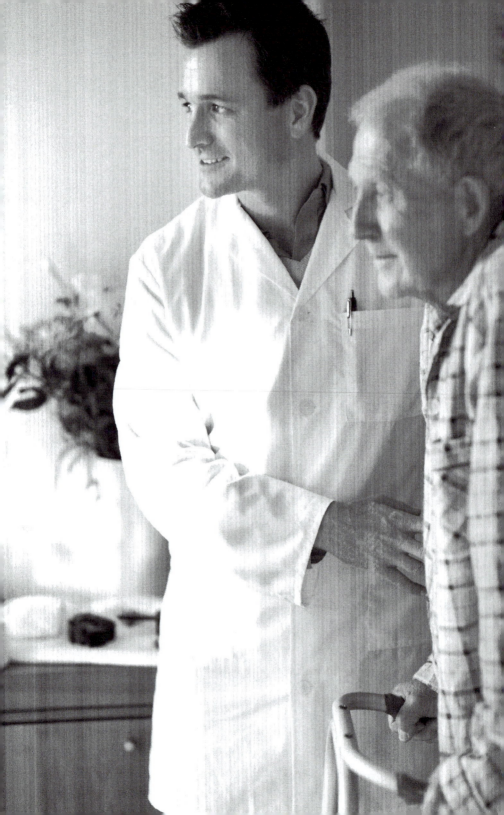

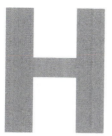

Humanity

Injustice anywhere is a threat to justice everywhere.

Martin Luther King Jr

A great leader has many desirable traits, amongst which is the ability to remain focused and driven but also being able to combine this with the ability to show compassion, kindness, fairness and empathy. In essence, an effective leader is able to demonstrate humanity. Humanity involves the understanding and expression of many different emotions. To act humanely towards others would seem to the majority a natural act. However, to act humanely effectively, particularly within leadership, requires a certain degree of skill and time to be able to really listen, understand and act upon others' feelings. If you are able to commit time to listening and then act humanely upon the things you hear, you will ultimately perform much more effectively as a leader. Those leaders who choose to ignore humanity within their working life may not progress with ease. To act without regard for others' feelings or emotions will lead to bad feeling towards you and your viewpoint and most importantly you may lose the respect of your team or organisation and even external stakeholders.

One of the more important components of humanity is the ability to show empathy and this is an essential building block for developing competence within any leadership style. Goleman et al. stated that 'leaders with empathy are able to attune to a wide range of emotional signals, letting them sense the felt, but unspoken, emotions in a person or group.'[27] Such leaders listen attentively and can grasp the other person's perspective. 'Empathy makes a leader able to get along well with people of diverse backgrounds or from other cultures.'[28] As this statement suggests, in order to achieve empathy and in turn to be able to act with humanity you must have the ability to listen attentively. Active listening involves tuning into verbal and non-verbal communication and taking a genuine interest in others. Once you have consciously listened, you can then begin the process of understanding and being able to gain insight into another person's thoughts or emotions. An empathetic leader is generally respected and well thought of and as such has significant influence over their staff, which results in a more productive and effective team.

Often leaders find themselves having to deal with situations where emotions run high and staff or patients can feel uneasy or distressed. Leaders may find themselves in a position where they have to manage a difficult situation or discipline a member of staff or embark upon complicated contract negotiations. Within these situations leaders should be mindful of the need to stay in control, but they must also be able to display empathy without inflaming emotions further. When the former Mayor of New York was asked to speculate on the number of deaths that were caused by the terrorist attack on the World Trade Center in September 2001, he answered with thought and compassion. He stated that 'whatever the final count, it would be more than any of us can bear.'[29] This is an excellent example of a strong and accomplished leader

27 Goleman, D., Boyatzis, R. and McKee, A. *Primal Leadership: Realizing the Power of Emotional Intelligence*, Harvard Business School Publishing, Boston, MA, 2002.
28 www.leadershape.biz
29 Goodwin, N. *Leadership in Health Care: A European Perspective*, Routledge Health Management Series, Routledge, London and New York, 2006, p103.

showing compassion without fuelling further negative emotions.

Empathy is most often the trait that needs to be developed in leaders, and as such Leadershape[30] has created a tool to test empathy in behavioural traits. Consider the following traits:

- I listen attentively to what people say.

- I demonstrate an awareness of how others are feeling.

- I accurately identify the underlying causes of the other person's perspective.

- I express an understanding of the other person's perspective.

If you can display these traits within your leadership style then you are considered to be able to demonstrate empathy effectively.

Another component of humanity is the ability to show compassion, which is defined as 'a strong feeling of understanding, pity or sympathy for the sufferings of others'.[31] To experience or deliver true compassion within the world of business, even in healthcare, is quite rare as it is sometimes seen as a weakness amongst hard-nosed business leaders. In actual fact, to show true compassion requires an individual to draw upon their inner strength, courage and power. Within healthcare organisations, displays of compassion will be demonstrated more readily and will generally not be considered a weakness. A healthcare leader by their very nature should have a natural propensity to show compassion as this is one of the qualities that links so many healthcare workers at all levels. You should, however, be careful not to confuse compassion with sympathy.

---

30 www.leadershape.biz
31 Manser, M. *The Heinemann English Dictionary*, 5th edition, Heinemann, Oxford, 2001.

'Compassion is a blend of fairness, kindness, gentleness, honesty, respect, courage and love.'[32]

The opportunity to demonstrate humanity will arise throughout your role as a leader and you should strive to incorporate humanity within all of your actions. A humane leader will be able to sense how their staff are feeling or how they are doing; they will care about their staff; and they will be able to react sensitively to their staff. Displaying all these qualities means a humane leader is considered by those that they lead to be understanding, genuine and trustworthy.
All of these resulting opinions of you as a leader will cause your team to be more willing to work with you to achieve your goals as your emotional self encourages them to trust your opinion and your leadership skills as a whole. Indeed, it is sometimes said that some human competencies that make up humanity, such as self-awareness, self-discipline, compassion and empathy, are of a greater significance than traditional intelligence when it comes to working effectively as a leader.

Taking humanity forward

▌ Reflect upon the empathy traits described in Leadershape. Assess yourself against these statements and consider ways in which you may behave more humanely within your leadership role.

▌ Read Goleman, Bryatzis and Mekee, *Primal Leadership: Realizing the Power of Emotional Intelligence,* as detailed in the Further reading list.

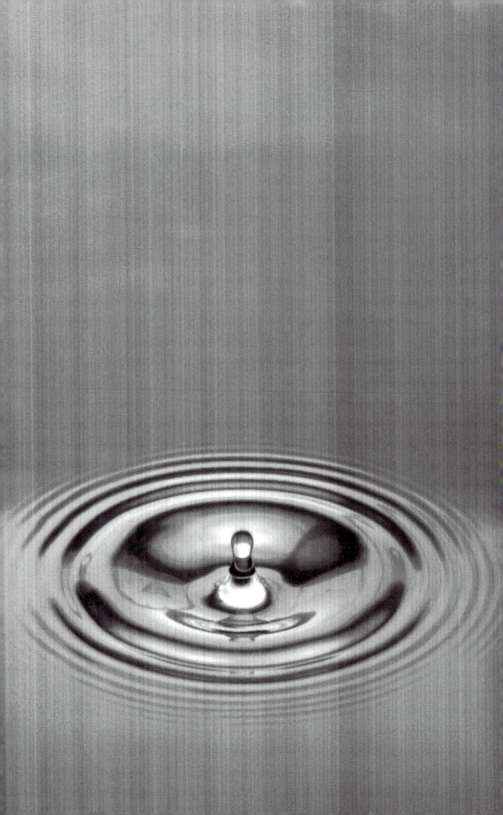

Influence

The final test of a leader is that he leaves behind him in other men the conviction and will to carry on.

Walter J Lippmann

nfluence is a form of persuasion: it's about persuading another individual or a group of individuals to adopt a certain way of thinking, to change their behaviour or to re-prioritise what they believe to be important. There are many forms of persuasion. You can persuade an individual to change their behaviour through dictatorial leadership, through physical or mental abuse, or through fear of the consequences of not conforming. Influence, however, is a gentle, clear and consistent persuasive approach. Influence is about applying fresh and creative non-threatening approaches to a contemporary situation, in order to effect change.[33] And if used correctly, influence should be used to change behaviours in order to better a team or organisation. It shouldn't be used to push forward personal agendas or secure individual promotions. Let's look at an example below.

John Woolman was an American Quaker who lived throughout the middle years of the 18th century. He was responsible for almost singlehandedly ridding the Religious Society of Friends (Quakers) of slaves. He devoted 30 years of his life to this cause, travelling from Quaker household to Quaker household to speak to slave owners. He used a

33 Greenleaf, R.F. *Servant Leadership: A Journey into the Nature of Legitimate Power and Greatness*, Paulist Press, New York, 2002, p23.

unique method of gentle, clear and persistent questioning and conversation to influence the slave owners' behaviour, enabling them to see that their actions were wrong, and that society would function in a more sustainable and just way if their behaviours changed. John Woolman was successful in his mission, with the Quakers becoming the first religious group to collectively renounce slavery.[34]

Influence is such an important leadership skill. To have the ability to influence the agendas of others, to change behaviours, to implement change *and* to have gained the support and enthusiasm of your audience (your 'influencees', if you like) is extremely powerful. It enables you to provide direction with minimal confrontation; and this can lead to a successful and cutting-edge organisation.

There are a number of different leadership styles in existence, and terminology for these styles varies depending on the book you're reading or the individual you're listening to. All styles, however, pull on the use of persuasion or influence to implement action or change and to push forward an agenda. Servant leadership, a term coined by Robert Greenleaf, is a popular contemporary concept in the world of leadership theory, and a leadership style that clearly highlights the power and importance of the skill of influencing.

In general terms, servant leadership is about leaders ensuring that other people's highest priority needs are being served; supporting individual agendas, and working for the overall benefit of the organisation as a whole. It can be difficult to reconcile these two almost juxtaposed terms, leader and servant. But as Blanchard states, ultimately leadership encompasses two roles – visionary and implementation.[35]

34 See note 33, p42–43.
35 Blanchard, K. *Leading at a Higher Level*, FT Prentice Hall, Pearson, Harlow, 2007, p248.

'The visionary role is the leadership aspect of servant leadership', whereas 'implementation is where the servant aspect of servant leadership comes into play'.[36] As a leader, you will have your vision and the vision of the organisation at the heart of your strategic aims. This vision may focus on improving patient care, on excelling in clinical research, on providing an excellent teaching environment, or on developing cutting-edge service delivery. Implementing this vision is where a servant leadership style appears to drive success. By focusing on the immediate needs and priorities of staff and of employers, by gaining their trust and respect, and respecting their agendas, you can use a consistent and persistent influential approach to drive change and meet your overarching vision.

So how can you put all this into practice? How can you actually *be* influential? Becoming a successful influencer is a skill that requires time and practice to master, and you need to have armour that incorporates an adaptable personal style and knowledge to successfully influence behaviours. The table below outlines the detail of that all-important armour.

Armour type	Correlating armour detail
Personal style	The ability to be an authentic leader
	Supportive and positive relationships with employers, peers and employees
	The ability to articulate and speak with passion and conviction
	Appropriate dress for your audience or 'influencees'

36 Blanchard, K. *Leading at a Higher Level*, FT Prentice Hall, Pearson, Harlow, 2007, p248.

Armour type	Correlating armour detail
Knowledge	Taking the time to do your homework! Knowing who to approach prior to a decision being made to ensure that your thoughts and agendas are fully considered
	Confident networking
	Understanding internal and external politics and being organisationally astute, and using this knowledge to gain support for your agenda

As a leader, you want and need to successfully implement your aims and vision, and the overarching vision of the organisation. To do so requires the support, energy and enthusiasm of your superiors, peers and employees. Gaining their support and commitment involves influencing their thoughts and often persuading them to change current practice. To influence others in this way you need sufficient armour of skills and knowledge that, if used correctly, will enable the realisation of your aims and visions.

Taking influence forward

▎ Do a self-assessment of your 'armour to influence' using the table above.

▎ Study the work of Robert Greenleaf (servant leadership) and reflect on the principles he exposes in relation to your own practice.

▎ Identify an opportunity to influence (positively) a situation in your organisation and use this as a learning opportunity.

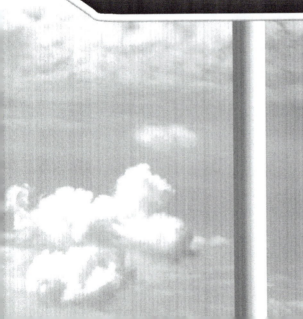

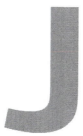

Judgement

Management is doing things right; leadership is doing the right things.

Peter F. Drucker

M aking judgements is something we all do frequently throughout our working day; whether it be in clinical diagnostics, to evaluate others' opinions or to draw conclusions from an article that we have read, it is an unavoidable occurrence. For some, making a judgement and basing decisions around that judgement is a behaviour that comes quite naturally. If an individual has a preconceived and definite viewpoint around a subject, then a judgement based on that subject may come naturally and almost without thought. However, also within this group of individuals are those who make judgements and decisions with ease but do so because they do not fully analyse the consequences or indeed the factors influencing their judgement. There are others, however, for whom making that initial judgement can be an arduous task and as a result there may be a delay in decision making. Whether it is an easy or a painstaking exercise, all judgements should always be made as a result of a well thought out process and not purely based on intuition or instinct; although it is certainly true that experience in similar situations over a period of time influences our judgements and the power of judgement making. In addition to making the conscious effort to think through your judgements you should also make a conscious effort to make a timely decision. There is no benefit from analysing a situation 'to death' but then being unable to make the step to draw a conclusion from your analysis.

Making good judgements and sound decisions as a result of these appraisals is imperative for a leader to be effective and to ensure that they are respected by their team and their boss. A successful leader will make timely and appropriate judgements using a certain degree of critical thinking. 'Critical thinking is the discipline of rigorously and skilfully using information, experience, observation and reasoning to guide your decisions, actions and beliefs.'[37] There are clear risks in making a judgement without the use of such critical thinking; these include making incorrect assumptions to base your decision upon and letting emotions unnecessarily influence your decisions. The presence of poor judgement, which suggests a lack of critical thinking, can ultimately lead to failure as a leader and the failure of a team. Healthcare leaders who have clinical backgrounds may be able to adapt their expert clinical critical thinking skills to leadership.

Within healthcare and the public sector as a whole there are definite complications that arise with respect to making judgements, particularly when they involve large budgets or when the resulting decisions will have direct effects on patient care. When making these difficult judgements, leaders should always use critical thinking to analyse all possible outcomes and effects and should always consider them in light of their stance as healthcare leaders and within the ideals of the healthcare system within which they work. This relates to the concept of authenticity; being true to yourself as a healthcare leader and your values will ultimately guide you through the decision making process. 'All decisions, big and small, should be consistent with the overall vision and direction that the organisation is

---

37 www.mindtools.com

headed.'[38] If this vision is clear when judgements are being made and they are made to steer towards that vision, then it becomes easier to make the relevant decisions without having to repeatedly question yourself and without having to seek approval from others.

If you apply the process of critical thinking then you should be confident that the judgements you have made are indeed correct for that time and place. It is inevitable, however, that as circumstances change and unexpected situations arise, your original judgement may become inappropriate and may need to change. As a good leader you should be prepared to accept that your judgements may require adjustment as such changes occur. If judgements are inappropriate due to the fact that the assumptions used to make them have changed, then they are not poor judgements in themselves. It is, though, poor judgement not to be flexible enough to rethink your decision and if necessary take a step backwards in terms of your original choices.

As a leader you will be required to make judgements on a whole range of ideas, people and processes. An effective leader will always approach a judgement with an open mind and, whilst working within the realms of authenticity, should always endeavour to consider all variations of arguments for and against, and should be open to considering other people's judgements. Often it is your team who will be able to provide the most valuable viewpoints with regard to the judgements that you have to make. A nurse working within a busy ward will have a far more realistic idea than anyone else of how policy changes could be implemented to resolve the pressures within that ward. Judgements, therefore, should be made not only by considering the impact on others but also by consulting others on their potential impact.

38 Barker, A.M., Sullivan, D.T. and Emery, M.J. *Leadership Competencies for Clinical Managers: The Renaissance of Transformational Leadership*, Jones and Bartlett, London, 2005, p132.

Taking judgement forward

▌ Read Browne, M.N. and Keeley, S.M. *Asking the Right Questions: A Guide to Critical Thinking*, 9th edition, Pearson, Harlow, 2009.

▌ Reflect upon a judgement you recently made that resulted in an improvement in patient care. What made this right? What influenced you?

▌ Reflect upon a judgement you regard as poor that you or another leader made. What happened and what might you learn from reflecting upon this situation?

[leadership]

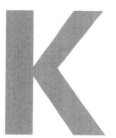

Knowledge

Education is the mother of leadership.

Wendell Willkie

Knowledge comes in many guises. It can be defined as information, facts, data, skill, education and intelligence. At the same time, knowledge is intrinsically related to wisdom, understanding, awareness and experience. Blanchard goes one step further and defines knowledge as 'going beyond merely acquiring information; it means actually learning from that information and applying that knowledge to new situations'.[39] So, knowledge isn't only about academia, education and clinical learning – it is much broader than that.

As a leader, there are several 'types' of knowledge that you need to ascertain, develop and utilise:

- clinical knowledge;
- leadership knowledge;
- current affairs.

Clinical knowledge

Clinical knowledge is almost self-explanatory; it involves keeping your professional practice and knowledge base up-to-date by building up wisdom, and growing your

39 Blanchard, K. *Leading at a Higher Level*, FT Prentice Hall, Pearson, Harlow, 2007, p77.

clinical expertise by using current clinical knowledge to learn about new clinical arenas. This involves proactively engaging in the clinical practices of frontline staff; how do they care for their patients? What research are they undertaking? What conclusions are they deriving? It also involves undertaking your own research; ensuring that you are reading role-specific publications, research papers, news items. Remember that as you grow and develop as a leader, and the remit of your role grows, so the clinical field in which you need to take an interest widens. You may have initially specialised as a Respiratory Nurse, then progressed to lead the Specialised Medicine team, and then advanced to lead the entire Medicine team. As your role grew, so did the number of clinical areas for which you took responsibility. And so, by default, your clinical knowledge base should grow and develop to encompass these new areas. Of course this can be daunting and some view this accelerated expansion of knowledge as often being impractical to achieve. For example, when I took up the chief nurse post at the Royal Marsden back in 1998, staff were at first perplexed by my appointment. Why? Well, because I had no prior knowledge or experience of working in a cancer service. I did, however, have extensive nursing and managerial experience, both of which I was able to use effectively to make strategic decisions outside of my specialty knowledge base. I knew the right questions to ask, I knew where to research cancer-specific information and I knew what information would set my internal alarm bells ringing ... and what aspects of the service to worry about. Building on and pulling from my initial clinical knowledge base enabled me to lead and develop new specialty and service areas.

Learning is of course an ongoing task: the key is to expand your knowledge base over time, incorporating new research areas, new practices, and new ways of working as you go along. Tom Peters, in his book *Re-imagine!,* makes a bold but truthful statement when he states that 'Leaders are great learners.'[40] He goes on to say that 'the best (and brightest) consultant I worked with in seven years at McKinsey had, I thought, one True Secret: he fearlessly and invariably asked … WHY? Effective leading = asking WHY? At least a dozen times a day.'[41] This definition of leading effectively by asking Why? can be applied to clinical, leadership and current affairs learning.

Leadership knowledge

There is a common misconception that 'leading' is a skill that just 'comes' to people; that once individuals have reached a particular 'level' within their professional career, or once they have gained a certain amount of clinical knowledge, that they will just become successful leaders. Unfortunately this isn't quite true! As with all skills and aptitudes, leading successfully requires the acquisition of knowledge, an understanding of how to use this knowledge, time to put these acquired skills into practice, reflection on how well-developed your leadership skills are, and a realignment of your skills based on continued self-assessment and continued learning. Becoming a talented neurosurgeon does not automatically make you a decent leader. Becoming a leader is a talent in its own right.

Evidence-based practice knowledge can be powerful and can be used to cement your personal presence, influence change and help you achieve desired outcomes. For those with a clinical background, the concept of evidence-based practice is well understood. But how does this knowledge help support your growth as a leader? In the same way that clinical practice is strongly grounded in the evidence of 'what

40 Peters, T. *Re-imagine! Business Excellence in a Disruptive Age*, Dorling Kindersley, London, 2003, p77.
41 See note above.

has been proven before', leadership practice should pull on evidence of successful working. This knowledge type is often overlooked by managers and non-clinical leaders, and is an area of expertise within which clinical leaders can excel. Taking the time to research and learn about evidence-based leadership practice can add further weight to your personal presence. Learning, for example, that comprehensive and timely appraisals have proven to have a positive impact on mortality rates can help you convince your colleagues to place a greater emphasis on staff development. In the same way, using evidence-based practice to support your argument that service-level financial reporting will empower frontline staff is impressive, convincing and powerful. This level of knowledge drives results, establishes trust, and helps define you as a leader. Effectively using external leadership knowledge has the same impact.

You can obtain additional leadership knowledge from a variety of areas. There are of course resource books (such as this one) that provide practical information and advice about what it means to be a leader. There are courses and seminars that teach you about common leadership themes, and provide face-to-face opportunities for you to 'practise' your leadership technique. You can also learn a lot from those around you. By watching other people's leadership style you can start to make decisions about how you want your leadership style or approach to be. Having a self-reflective attitude is also important to developing an effective leadership style. Undertaking a 360-degree appraisal takes guts; you have to have sufficient confidence in your ability to use the outcome effectively to put yourself under that level of scrutiny. However, appraisals of this kind are a constructive experience as they provide you with the opportunity to benchmark your own skills and abilities against those required to successfully carry out your role. All of these learning options provide crucial leadership

knowledge ... your success as a leader will depend upon
how well you utilise this knowledge, and apply it to your
own leadership style.

Current affairs

Knowledge is everywhere! There are so many subject areas
to learn about, to have an opinion on, and to explore. And as
your knowledge base grows, you find links appear from one
subject area to another; information that initially impacts
on one particular subject arena ends up affecting others.
The national and international political agenda impacts
on healthcare, and the direction in which you lead your
team or department. Environmental issues impact on your
list of service development priorities for the year. National
legal changes affect how you interact with staff, population
demographics change the type of patients you work with on
a daily basis – current affairs matter!

As a leader, you need a wide appreciation of the world at
large. Healthcare organisations, like all other organisations,
need knowledge of political agendas, environmental and
economical issues, and 'customer' demographics to survive,
or at least function successfully. The vast majority of patients
in developed countries are now able to access information
about their health conditions and about their healthcare
rights before even setting foot inside a hospital. Staff need
to be aware of this, and change the way that they respond
to patient questions and queries to accommodate this
ever-growing patient knowledge. Blanchard states that 'high
performing organisations seek knowledge by constantly
scanning the environment, checking the pulse of their
customers, tracking their competition, surveying the market,
and following global events'.[42] The same principles apply

42 Blanchard, K. *Leading at a Higher Level*, FT Prentice Hall, Pearson, Harlow,
2007, p77.

to healthcare leadership. You can't gain this knowledge by purely focusing on your particular team, specialty, interest or even healthcare in general. You have to look wider than these parameters, and seek knowledge of contemporary affairs that matter.

Taking knowledge forward

▌ Read a broadsheet newspaper at least once a day.

▌ Assess the impact on the public of national health-related issues, through your knowledge of current affairs.

▌ Read three evidence-based papers that provide information on relevant practices (clinical or leadership) which you could apply to your current role.

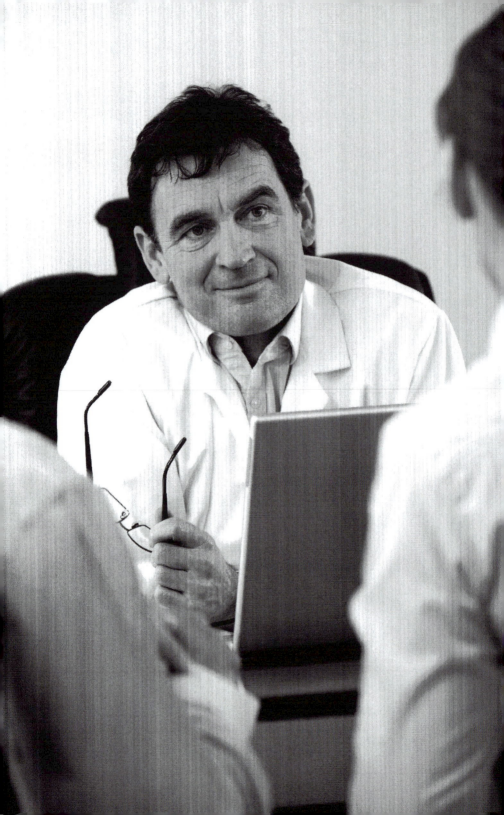

Listening

Many attempts to communicate are nullified by saying too much.

Robert Greenleaf

t is an important leadership skill to be able to communicate clearly with others. It is essential that you are able to convey information to others in an effective manner but it is equally important that you are able to receive information from others and therefore vital that you are able to listen effectively. Many people assume that they have the ability to listen well, however, the perception you have of your ability to listen may not be accurate as there is a definite skill to listening and it is not something that everyone is naturally good at, although they may think they are. 'Listening is harder than most people realise because it is an acquired skill just like reading or writing.'[43] If you improve your listening ability you can greatly improve your leadership skills.

Manny Steil, the CEO of Communication Development Inc., teaches the basics of listening concepts and divides the act of listening into four areas that all need to be developed. These are:

▌ **Sensing** – the ability to hear the words.

▌ **Interpretation** – being able to understand the words.

---

43 Manny Steil, CEO of Communication Development Inc., www.techrepublic.com/article/enhance-your-listening-skills-and-your-management-success/5054191

▍ **Evaluation** – the ability to accept or reject the words.

▍ **Responding** – taking a final action that results from the conversation.

There are many reasons why individuals struggle with the first area of actually hearing the words. Sometimes this is caused by physical distractions, such as background noise from other people or equipment. Sometimes the listener may be distracted by other thoughts or emotions and therefore is unable to pay attention. To be an effective listener you should always be aware of how your emotions can impair your ability to listen and to understand what is being said. A good listener should always try to focus on a conversation and deflect any alternative thoughts, emotions or background distractions as it is their responsibility to ensure that they understand what has been said. Focusing can also be a problem when the subject matter being discussed seems tedious or irrelevant. This causes individuals to adopt the skill of selective listening; 'some people listen well on subjects close to their heart, but on other topics, they don't hear a thing'.[44]

Once you have heard the words you should then take the time to interpret, evaluate and respond to them. This should be a considered process; you should never respond instantly without thinking through exactly what you have just heard. To absorb, interpret and evaluate the information that is being given to you can take time. It is often useful to demonstrate that you are actively processing information by asking direct questions of the speaker or by simply looking interested and acknowledging key points. Summarising key points and asking questions confirms that you have understood the information and allows you to consolidate it in your mind. 'Depending on the study being quoted, we remember a

44 See note 43.

dismal 25–50 per cent of what we hear.'[45] This means that for every 10 minutes of conversation we only really hear about 2½–5 minutes of it. Therefore to paraphrase what has been said will help us to retain more of the conversation.

Traits that demonstrate that an individual has bad listening habits are described in the book *Listen Up* by Barker and Watson.[46] These traits can include:

▌ interrupting the speaker;

▌ not looking at the speaker;

▌ rushing the speaker;

▌ showing interest in something else;

▌ getting ahead of the speaker and finishing their sentences;

▌ not responding to questions posed by the speaker;

▌ forgetting what has been asked of you;

▌ asking too many questions in regard to irrelevant details.

If you can recognise any of the above traits in your behaviour then you should endeavour to improve your listening skills.

Listening effectively has many benefits; you will not only obtain more information from the people you lead but you will also increase their trust in you as you prove to them that you are listening to their opinions and requests. In addition, a leader that listens will learn more about the individuals they are leading and will then be better equipped to understand how to motivate their team. In

45 www.mindtools.com
46 Barker, L. and Watson, K. *Listen Up: How to Improve Relationships, Reduce Stress and Be More Productive by Using the Power of Listening*, Macmillan Audio, New York, 2000.

turn this will inspire a higher level of commitment in the individuals working with and for them. 'A study of managers and employees in a hospital system found that listening explained 40 per cent of the variance in leadership.'[47] Therefore to be seen as a good leader you should be known as a good listener. This is a skill that must be worked upon: 'Good communication skills require a high level of self awareness. By understanding your personal style of communicating you will go a long way towards creating good and lasting impressions with others.'[48] Once you can understand the listening skills you possess and become aware of those you need to improve, you will be able to work towards becoming an effective listener and ultimately the rewards for this will be many.

As a leader you don't just need to be a good listener, you need people to listen to you, especially those who report to you and those above you in the hierarchy. A key part of 'managing upwards' is ensuring that your 'boss' listens to you. It is therefore important to choose your moment when you need to share something with your boss. Do so at a time when they can focus on you, when they are not busy with something else or dashing to a meeting; for example, 5pm on a Friday, the day they are going on holiday or when they are about to go into an important board meeting is not a time to bother them!

If your boss seems distracted when you are about to speak with them, you can politely say that you would like to discuss 'x' issue but will speak to them at a time when they are not so busy.

47 www.wright.edu
48 www.mindtools.com

Taking listening forward

▌ Self-evaluate your own listening skills using the framework provided in *Listen Up*.

▌ Reflect upon a situation in which you failed to listen properly. Why? What happened? What would you have done differently?

▌ Reflect upon ways in which you can ensure optimal conditions for being listened to.

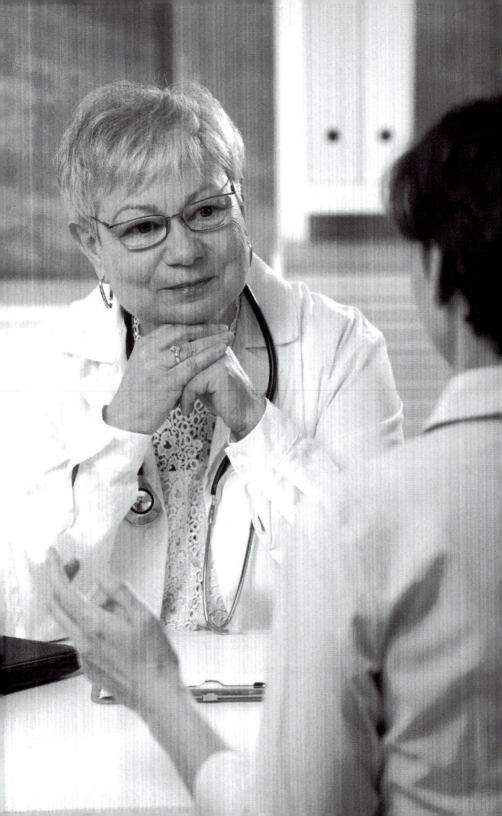

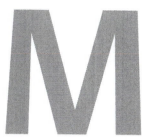

Mentorship

A leader has the vision and conviction that a dream can be achieved. He inspires the power and energy to get it done.

Ralph Nader

The concepts of mentorship and coaching are often confused as being much the same thing. Whilst they share similar traits they are different, with mentorship relating much more to an individual's personal development and career development throughout their life, and helping 'to progress individual careers by increasing personal self-esteem and satisfaction and helping individuals use their intelligence more fully to make a contribution to personal and organisational success'.[49] Coaching, on the other hand, relates to an individual's confidence and aptitude whilst undertaking a specific role or job. It generally refers to 'training, that is guidance and feedback about specific efforts involved in a task, performance of a job, and handling of assignments. The broad field of coaching may include life planning, career counselling, health advice and training in specific skills.'[50] Both mentoring and watching, however, involve 'developing individuals and their capabilities through communication, feedback, encouragement and praise'.[51] As a leader, you should strive to provide, undertake and encourage

49 Goodwin, N. *Leadership in Health Care: A European Perspective*, Routledge Health Management Series, Routledge, London and New York, 2006, p164.
50 See note above.
51 Creative Nursing Management, *Leading an Empowered Organisation*, University of Leeds, Handout, 1994. (The organisation has since become Creative Health Care Management, **www.chcm.com**.)

both mentorship and coaching as and when this level of support and feedback is required. Whilst not everybody needs mentoring or coaching at all stages of their career, 'individuals may find it particularly helpful to have a mentor when they are at critical points in their career development'.[52]

There are of course key themes which are applicable to both mentorship and coaching. Any mentoring or coaching programme needs to have a clear focus, purpose or aim which is reviewed frequently. A mentor or coach should ideally be an individual who sits outside the mentee's (or mentoree's) organisation, and certainly shouldn't be the mentee's line manager (however, it is recognised that a competent line manager will, as a matter of course, fulfil some of the responsibilities of a mentor).[53] Whilst an individual's line manager will be task-orientated, their mentor or coach should be focused on the mentee's overall well-being and development as a person – taking an interest in their progress, acting as a sounding board for their ideas and concerns, and being a guide by 'showing them the ropes' of the job.[54] A line management relationship is often built on respect. A mentoring or coaching relationship should be built on trust.

Both mentors and mentees have responsibilities that they must fulfil if the mentoring or coaching programmes are to be productive and beneficial. For mentors, these responsibilities revolve around the requirement to possess certain skills or qualities that need to be utilised in a mentoring programme. These include:

▌ objectivity;

▌ a positive attitude towards developing others;

52 The Centre for the Development of Nursing Policy and Practice, *Mentoring*, University of Leeds, Handout, undated. (The centre is now called Centre for Innovation in Health Management, **www.cihm.leeds.ac.uk**.)
53 See note above.
54 See note 52.

▌ integrity;

▌ authenticity;

▌ balanced judgement;

▌ patience;

▌ openness to ideas;

▌ an ability to listen;

▌ a willingness to share information;

▌ an ability to provide constructive feedback.[55]

For mentees, responsibilities are more task-orientated and include:

▌ preparing for meetings with mentor;

▌ attending meetings with mentor and adhering to the agreed programme timetable;

▌ taking responsibility for learning and development;

▌ respecting the confidentiality of the relationship with their mentor.[56]

As a leader, encouraging a mentoring or coaching programme that will develop your employees is key to your role. But obviously not everyone can complete this type of programme; your decision as to who you should encourage to undertake this development has to be targeted. Many people struggle with the idea of prioritising certain individuals for career development, but it's never practical for everyone to complete such programmes all the time, and so for the benefit of the organisation you have to prioritise somehow! There are three principal reasons for

---

55 The Centre for the Development of Nursing Policy and Practice, *Mentoring*, University of Leeds, Handout, undated.
56 See note above.

targeting or encouraging certain individuals to develop in
this way:

1 They require a highly supportive and highly directive
leadership approach to fulfil their role.

2 They require the confidence and empowerment to believe
that they are worthy of career development.

3 They are a 'tall poppy' (i.e. an individual whose potential
for development and a future leadership role makes them
stand out from the crowd).

Those requiring a supportive approach

Think back to when you were learning to ride a bike.
Initially you were so excited you could barely sleep, even
though you had no idea how to actually ride the bike. You
were a classic enthusiastic beginner who required some
direction – the sort of direction a line manager provides for
their staff.

Now think about the first time (and second, third and
fourth!) you fell off your bike. As you hit the pavement you
probably wondered why you wanted to learn to ride a bike
in the first place. You were a bit of a disillusioned learner,
requiring a lot of support and praise, but clear direction from
your teacher. Here you benefited from supportive coaching
as well as directive line management.[57]

Employees are the same. At times when they require
both supportive and directive leadership, it makes sense
to encourage them to enter into a mentoring or coaching
programme.

57 Blanchard, K. *Leading at a Higher Level*, FT Prentice Hall, Pearson, Harlow,
2007, p90.

Those requiring empowerment

All leaders have a responsibility to strive for equality
and diversity with their people, and whilst there are now
policies, guidelines and often whole teams dedicated to
encouraging and enforcing equality and diversity in the
workplace, this doesn't mean that minority groups feel
empowered to progress or develop their careers. Encouraging
minority groups to apply for job promotions, to undertake
training, and to develop their careers through mentorship
helps empower, boosts confidence and supports diversity
across your organisation.

Those who are 'tall poppies'

'Tall poppies' are individuals who excel in their roles, or
who possess the skills and qualities to be high achievers.
They may be very different to you – they may possess
different mannerisms, qualities, beliefs and skills – but
nonetheless, they are still high achievers. These are
the individuals you look for at interview. They are the
candidates that could, for example, take over your role when
you leave – they are the individuals you think about when
completing your succession planning. For the benefit of the
organisation, these are the individuals you prioritise for
career development, and who you encourage to complete
beneficial mentorship programmes.

Taking mentorship forward

▌ If you don't already have one, seek your boss's support to enable you to have a mentor or coach.

▌ After appropriate development, offer your services as a mentor/ coach to other people.

▌ Privately, identify 'tall poppies' in your team, department or organisation. What can you do to help develop them?

▌ Take active and positive steps to encourage equality and diversity in leaders with whom you work and/or those you mentor.

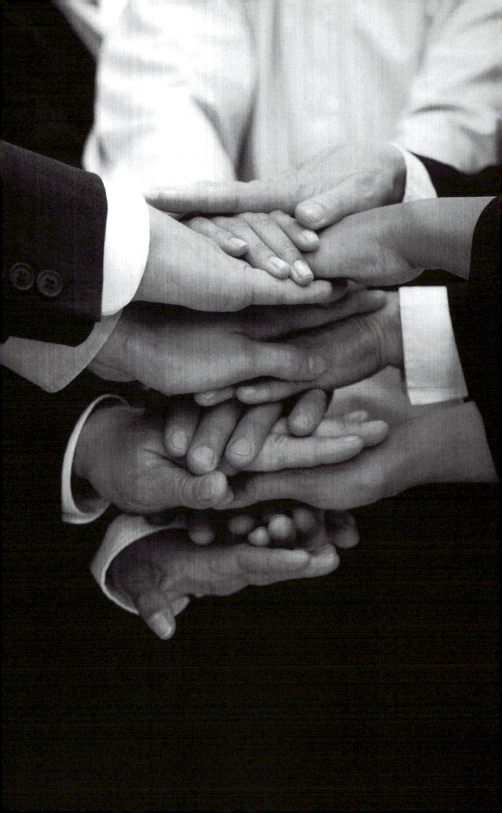

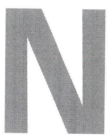

Networking

You cannot shake hands with a clenched fist.

Golda Meir

Using the principles of servant leadership, one of the key aims of networking in healthcare is to successfully associate oneself with a diverse group of individuals who can provide support, feedback, access to resources, information, and collaborative projects or research which will result in an improved service provision for staff and patients. A secondary aim may be more personal and related to career development, for example. Networking can sometimes mistakenly be perceived as the process by which an individual attempts to manipulate a group of people for the sole purpose of self-promotion or egotistical gain. For networking to deliver a positive outcome it must be a focused and proactive endeavour, and requires give and take from all parties involved. A good networker will set aside dedicated time on a regular basis to interact with people in their networks, which can at times be a difficult commitment to stick to when considering the prioritisation of workloads. Networking 'demands a readiness to contribute when you cannot be sure you will receive a full return on your investment'.[58] However, good networking can save you time! For example, using someone in your network to provide copies of business cases or research proposals they have used successfully saves you 'reinventing the wheel'.

58 Leigh, A. *The Secrets of Success in Management: 20 Ways to Survive and Thrive*, Pearson, Harlow, 2009, p58.

Before attempting to network you must understand exactly what you wish to achieve from your networks. A strong network has the potential to provide enhanced power and political influence and can therefore push forward agendas much more readily and successfully than any autonomous individual. Setting a clearly defined goal will enable you to develop a focused strategy. The goal should not be self-serving but should reflect your desire to make a positive impact on your organisation and all those involved with its services, whether this be patients, staff or colleagues. Once you have decided upon your objective you should then go forward and identify any existing networks that you can tap into and also those that you can initiate and develop yourself. These might be professional associations, online professional groups or indeed committees that you are on. Identify people that will help you to achieve your aim; consider both what you are looking for and what you are prepared to offer to the network. Once you have identified your network you must then make the conscious effort to develop and maintain relationships.

The practical side of networking is something that does not always come easily. It involves a certain amount of bravery to initiate a relationship, either by making that first telephone call or by introducing yourself to a stranger in a crowd. In order that you make this initial contact a success, you must be prepared. Prepare a confident introductory sentence, which should be concise and informative. Remember that the potential to network can arise in a range of environments including conferences, meetings and even social events; therefore your opening statement should be adaptable to suit your audience. This introduction should clearly inform others of your name and what you do but it should then quickly turn the focus of the conversation back to the individual you are talking to. By doing this you can find out more about the person in front of you and you can then start to consider how they could fit into your network and also how you could work together to achieve each other's objectives. Once you have engaged in conversation it is vital that you make a conscious effort to listen and take in what people are saying to you. If you can pick up on just one key objective or statement you can use this to initiate a follow-up conversation or contact and thus begin the process of developing a networking relationship.

The second area in which you must be prepared is to ensure that you can provide a means of contacting each other again. You must therefore have readily available business cards, making sure that they detail up-to-date, full and correct contact information and, if possible, the design should in some way reflect who you are and what you stand for. You must also be ready to note down their contact details in case they are not quite so well prepared as you! You should always follow up with an email a few days later, even if it simply says, 'It was a pleasure to meet you.'

Once you have identified individuals and made the initial contact it is imperative that you then have an organised way to record the information you have obtained. Make informal notes after any contact but then ensure that these are translated into a more formal record, ideally within an electronic contacts database. Within this database you should record information such as names, titles, email addresses and phone numbers but also details of conversations and dates of any previous contact, whether this be a one-to-one interaction, a telephone call or an email. Keeping up-to-date records is good working practice in all areas and especially in this instance will make contacting individuals within your network considerably more time and labour efficient, a priority for any successful leader.

You must be tenacious in following up contacts and also in developing your networking skills. When considering the networks that you are part of, whether formal or informal, it must be remembered that in all circumstances they will constantly be changing and evolving; 'networks are not static – if we use them, they constantly expand, but if we neglect them, they will shrink.'[59] If you persist with networking and remain focused on your initial networking objectives then eventually your goals will be achieved; the art of networking will become second nature to you and networking will be a commonplace feature in your daily working life. The sign of a great networker is someone of whom you 'ask them a question and they instantly know someone, who knows someone, who might know the answer'.[60]

Taking networking forward

▌ Identify a professional issue that you need help with and find someone that can help you to resolve it.

▌ Start to develop an electronic database of your contacts, such as Microsoft Outlook.

▌ Join one of the large electronic professional networks such as Linked In (**www.linkedin.com**).

59 Institute of Management *Small Business Management*, 10th edition, Hodder & Stoughton, London, 1999, p135.
60 Leigh, A. *The Secrets of Success in Management: 20 Ways to Survive and Thrive*, Pearson, Harlow, 2009, p58.

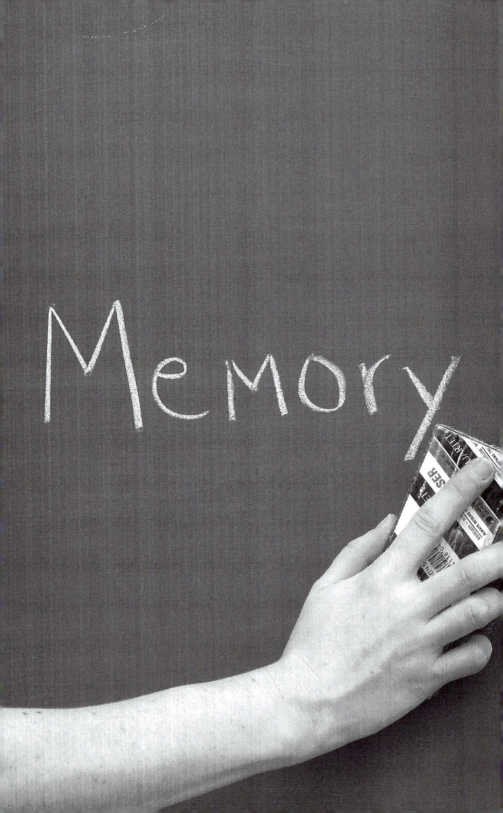

Organisational memory

Organisational effectiveness does not lie in that narrow minded concept called rationality. It lies in the blend of clearheaded logic and powerful intuition.

Henry Mintzberg

Organisational memory is a collection of all the factors that have ever influenced an organisation in making it what it is today. It is all the knowledge acquired, the information gained and lessons learnt. Organisational memory is invaluable when it comes to realising where the organisation has come from, determining where it should be going and, of course, the best way to get there. Reflecting on mistakes made, lessons learnt and success stories will provide a good basis for future decision making and planning processes. Using organisational memory in this way saves both time and energy and should push forward progress as individuals can avoid 'reinventing the wheel'. Using organisational memory is also a good way of embedding best practice within the foundations of a healthcare organisation. Organisational memory being used in this way has been defined as 'the ability of an organization to sustain new initiatives, to institutionalize the initiatives in the organization's standard operating procedures and to "routinize" the initiatives to make them a permanent component of the organization'.[61]

61 Virani, T., Lemieux-Charles, L., Davis, D.A. and Berta, W. 'Sustaining Change: Once Evidence-Based Practices Are Transferred, What Then?', *Longwoods Review*, 2009, Vol. 6, No. 4.

There is also another very important need for maintaining and using organisational memory and this relates to risk management and patient safety. If staff are not regularly reminded about the rationale behind specific organisational practices that have been developed as a result of serious untoward incidents that form part of organisational memory, then they may revert to old habits that compromise patient safety. For example, 'keeping the bed at the lowest level and leaving the side rail down will prevent a patient from climbing over the side rail, falling and seriously getting hurt'.[62] If a member of staff is not aware of the organisational memory surrounding this practice they may, in their ignorance, consider it to be an unnecessary action even though history suggests otherwise. There is a definite danger that without some element of organisational memory you can make the same clinical mistakes that have been made in the past, and which are usually avoidable multi-system failings.

Aspects of organisational memory (OM) are not always written down. OM can be purely a collection of others' memories of previous experiences. One way of understanding organisational memory therefore is to ask the appropriate questions from others and to proactively seek out information that is useful. Another way to familiarise yourself with organisational memory is by reading old policies, action plans and minutes from meetings. This way you are able to see a formal record of why certain things have been done and you will better be able to understand how processes have come into being or how a department structure has evolved and why. Without this knowledge you could end up undoing actions that have been put into place for a solid, historic, evidence-based reason. Another invaluable source of information with regard to organisational memory are long-term patients who

62 See note 61.

themselves will have seen changes in the management and care they receive. These are the individuals who are directly affected by the policies that you as a leader will implement, and if they have seen similar policies in the past they will have a very valid view of their success and could be able to prevent you repeating ineffective practices.

For new and less experienced leaders, it is essential that you draw upon the benefits that organisational memory provides. It would be foolish to completely ignore or not listen to the views and experiences of others who have been around for longer and who have seen evolution within the organisation. More experienced leaders may not necessarily have the best approaches for moving forward but they will certainly have some valuable memories of the past and as such you should take time to listen to their views and make your decisions based partly on their organisational memory.

Progress in healthcare globally is now so rapid and healthcare organisations evolve so quickly that organisational memory can be lost. This can happen as a result of organisations merging, departmental changes, structural changes, quick turnover of leaders, etc. All of these events are normally turbulent and will inevitably destroy some organisational memory. It is therefore important that organisational memory is respected and maintained despite the occurrence of potentially damaging events. 'For experiential learning to take place, companies and other institutions have to better manage their organizational memory (OM), the corporate equivalent of individual DNA.'[63] Successfully managing organisational memory and using an organisation's history in a positive way, as opposed to dwelling on the negatives of the past, will positively influence both the present and the future. The

---

63 Kransdorff, A. *Corporate DNA: Using Organizational Memory to Improve Poor Decision-making*, Gower, Farnham, 2006, p10.

positive way to look at the past is to accept that things may have previously failed and to then determine why they failed in order to avoid such repetition. A good leader should also hold the opinion that just because something has not previously been attempted it does not necessarily mean that it will now fail. Looking at historic positive experiences and appreciating the value of organisational memory will allow you as a leader to gain important knowledge and to apply evidence-based theory to your leadership practice.

Taking organisational memory forward

▌ Try to explore some of the historical roots of your organisation. Google may be a good place to start. Depending on where you work, you might even find books detailing aspects of the organisation's past. This research might help you to understand the situation (whether positive or negative) in your organisation, the services offered, the attitudes of staff and the public's perceptions.

▌ Review ways in which organisational memory is encouraged and enabled within your organisation, such as through minutes and papers.

▌ If you were suddenly and unexpectedly unable to come to work and/or communicate, what five aspects of organisational memory would it be vital for others to know about? List the five key areas and find practical ways of working the information about these areas into accessible, available and shareable media.

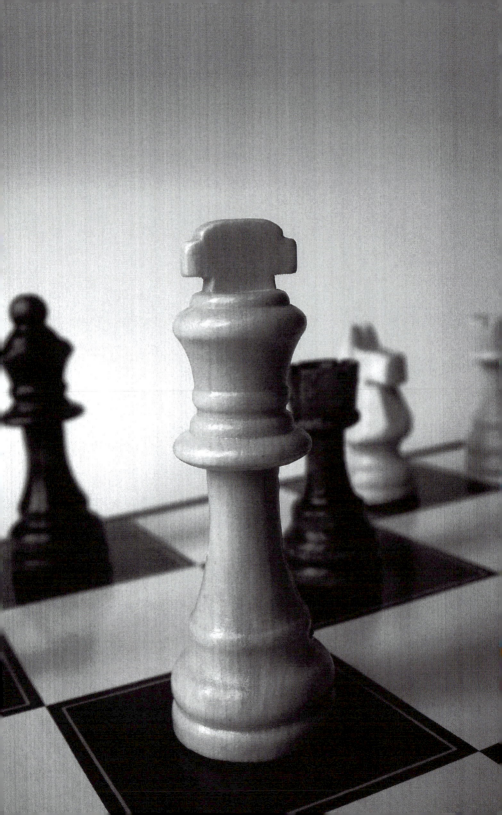

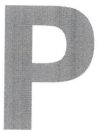

Power and politics

The price of greatness is responsibility.

Winston Churchill

Effective leadership requires the ability to be politically savvy, to recognise and respect organisational politics, to understand the importance of positional and personal power, and to use this understanding and recognition when establishing your own role within the hierarchy. Understanding the organisation that you're working in, understanding the local power struggles and having contemporary knowledge of the external factors that influence your organisation, specialty, directorate or team is very powerful and, used correctly, can help cement your position as a leader. As Charles Handy famously said, 'If we are to understand organisations we must understand the nature of power and influence, for they are the means by which the people of the organisation are linked to its purpose.'[64]

So knowledge is power! But more importantly, it is the ability to use this knowledge appropriately that builds great leaders. Leadership knowledge can be split into two different knowledge types – internal knowledge and external knowledge. Internal knowledge can be split again, into evidence-based knowledge and political knowledge, whereas external knowledge is concerned with current affairs, and

64 Handy, C. *Understanding Organizations*, 3rd edition, Penguin, London, 1985, p118.

how these affect your purpose, role and remit (see figure below).

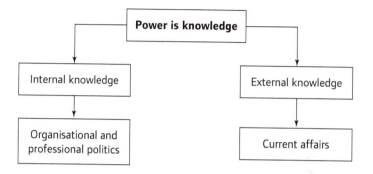

There seem to be two opposing schools of thought about organisational politics. One school ignores the impact of organisational politics, or tries to remove it through the advocacy of flat or matrix organisational structures. The belief is that by removing an obvious hierarchy, internal politics or the use of positional power can also be removed. In complete contrast, the second school of thought recognises and celebrates internal politics and power. It suggests that the use of internal politics is a constructive way to work with stakeholders, and states that through politics, individuals can value the many diverse and compelling agendas that are at work in all organisations today.[65]

Whether you view internal politics as a positive or a negative element of organisational working, it is very difficult to argue that internal politics don't exist, particularly within a healthcare setting, where a great mixture of professionals, academics, leaders and managers are brought together in one environment. How many times have you used an internal political viewpoint to get a desired result, be it

65 www.som.cranfield.ac.uk/som/p15254/Knowledge-Interchange/Hot-Topics/
General-Management/Gaining-Agreement-A-Constructive-Approach-to-Organisational-
Politics

clinical, financial or target-driven? How many times have you used the reputation of the organisation, the benefit of the patient, or the impact on the staff to secure additional funding, to improve a service, to change a clinical practice? In doing so you are not only acknowledging the existence of organisational politics, you are astutely using them too!

Internal politics are closely related to power. Within healthcare, hierarchical and professional structures are in place, and they should be respected. Ultimately, an Executive Director 'has authority because of his or her position within the organisation, which imparts power and enables [them] to influence others, whether they like it or not'.[66] Of course this ability to use power does not make them a great leader but nonetheless, in aspiring to be a great leader yourself, you need to respect those in positions of authority.[67] Openly displaying disrespectful behaviour or sharing negative opinions or gossip about those individuals who hold the power within your organisation may undermine your own position and power as a leader, and will display your political naiveté.

Don't forget, of course, that it isn't those individuals who sit at the top of the organisational and professional 'food chains' that possess all the power. Power can be found in two forms, positional (such as an Executive Director) and personal (i.e. someone who formally has little authority but who is highly influential, such as the CEO's secretary!). Perhaps the most overlooked group of powerful individuals in an organisation is the Personal Assistants or Secretaries. Keep them happy – at all costs! They make organisations tick and can make a leader's life either a pleasure or a nightmare. Using your knowledge of internal politics within an organisation to help

66 Gitlow, A. *Being the Boss: The Importance of Leadership and Power*, Business One Irwin, Homewood, IL, 1991.
67 Management Research Group, *Leadership Effectiveness Analysis*, Handout, 1998.

ground your personal presence and to successfully influence others is a key leadership skill. Ignoring or misusing this knowledge will undermine your personal presence, position and leadership abilities.

In a national survey of Australian executives, 95 per cent of interviewees stated that politics had an impact on the decisions made within their organisations. Furthermore, 87 per cent of interviewees said that 'organisational savvy' should be a required management competency.[68] The importance of political knowledge is clear. The removal of hierarchical structures will not remove the need to be politically astute to succeed as a leader within healthcare. Being organisationally savvy means understanding how to use internal politics, respecting power and authority, using authority as a resource for information, direction and decision-making,[69] and recognising the impact that external knowledge can have on your own leadership style.

Taking power and politics forward

▌ Study one of the texts referred to in this chapter.

▌ Through literature searching, identify a published evidence-based paper on an aspect of leadership practice that is relevant to you, your team or your organisation. The evidence-base for linking high appraisal rates and mortality rates in hospital is a good example. How could you utilise such evidence-based leadership in your practice?

▌ Identity three people in your organisation who have a high degree of personal power. How can you work with them differently to harness this power?

68 http://personaglobal.com/part_books_articles.aspx?id=2
69 See note 67.

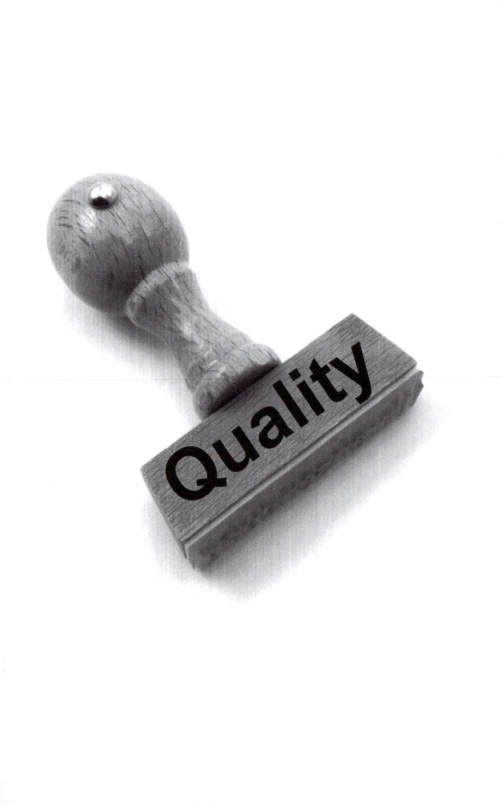

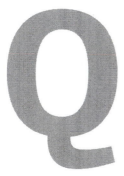

Quality assurance

Quality is never an accident; it is always the result of high intention, sincere effort, intelligent direction and skilful execution; it represents the wise choice of many alternatives.

Willa A. Foster

Quality standards are generally determined by the intended users of a service or those that commission or regulate it. Within healthcare the level of quality expected is to a degree defined by those using the service, such as patients or visitors to healthcare establishments. Quality assurance is normally sought through a set of activities that are intended to ensure that services satisfy customer needs and requirements in a systematic and reliable manner. This information can be collected through the use of patient experience surveys, using regulators' audits and by proactively seeking the views of others, via user groups, for example. There are other useful tools which can be used to pick up quality standards; these include key performance indicators (KPIs) and benchmarking against other organisations. All of these methods and more will lead to a certain level of quality assurance that should provide a level of service that allows for users to have confidence in their care providers and the leaders within the organisation. It is important to consider that not all users are the same and that their expectations and priorities for quality will vary greatly. As a leader therefore you should make every effort to ensure that you hear everyone's opinion and that all viewpoints are taken into consideration in planning quality standards. There have traditionally been certain groups who have not had their voice heard, including those with learning disabilities, mental health problems, ethnic minorities, and lesbian, gay, bisexual and transgender people, but as a leader it is your responsibility to seek out and work with their opinions.

Healthcare organisations have quality standards set at many levels. The government provides higher level quality assurance in the form of target setting and performance management. These higher level standards give a clear message to the end user of the quality that they should expect on a national level throughout the healthcare industry. Quality assurance can also be defined within individual organisations and within departments and these can be over and above the quality standards defined at a national level. To provide additional quality assurance in this way allows for leaders to work towards a local vision that is relevant to the demographic using their service. There is also the need for internal quality assurance, which involves more inward-looking processes to assess individual practices and to determine how you as a leader are meeting expectations and how your team are performing against your and their expectations.

The use of quality assurance within healthcare helps to improve the service provided and to enhance the organisation's profile. This is also achieved through clinical governance which directly impacts on quality assurance. Clinical governance is the system used to ensure high standards of patient care; the guidance provided should create an environment within which clinical excellence can flourish, thus once again leading to an improved service delivery and an enhanced organisational profile. As a healthcare leader, good clinical quality assurance should be what motivates you towards improving standards within your organisation. Improving clinical standards directly impacts on quality assurance for patients, and ultimately your aim as a leader is to ensure that patient care and patients' experience of your organisation are of the highest quality.

In England there is an independent regulator of healthcare organisations, the Care Quality Commission (CQC), which exists to ensure that those bodies are providing an acceptable level of care and that the care provided is quality assured.[70] There are similar regulators in Scotland, Wales and Northern Ireland. They all work closely with the UK-wide regulators of healthcare professionals such as the Nursing and Midwifery Council (NMC) and General Medical Council (GMC).

As a leader it is your responsibility to be knowledgeable of the quality assurance levels expected within your team and your organisation as a whole. It is your responsibility to listen to the views and opinions of those using the service you are providing, and if necessary it is your responsibility to apply improved quality assurance measures to meet the end users' requirements. Having listened and defined quality standards it is then also your job to lead on the delivery of these standards. Meeting targets, such as reducing waiting times or improving GP access, will not happen without a proactive lead implementing the necessary strategies required. However, sometimes quality assurance can feel like a purely bureaucratic process and for some it may seem as though the only reason for quality assurance is to chase government-set targets or to please senior management. As a leader, therefore, it is your role to ensure that you educate your team about the real need for and the purpose of quality assurance and to motivate them to embrace it in a positive manner. If the profile of quality assurance is approached positively by a group and led in a proactive way by an effective leader, then the team's efforts will result in a positive impact on patient care. Having motivated your team and successfully implemented quality assurance strategies it is then vital that you monitor performance against goals so that you are aware of the steps you have made and/or still need to make towards improving or indeed maintaining quality within your organisation.

Taking quality assurance forward

▌ Review and critique the quality specifications relevant to your area of practice, discipline or organisation. What one thing could you do as a leader to ensure a greater degree of compliance?

▌ Develop your thoughts, depending on your job role, now and in the future, on how you will better engage with some of the groups whose voices are heard less, as listed in the first paragraph of this chapter.

▌ Ensuring a high quality of work is everyone's responsibility. Define your specific responsibilities and include these in your objectives.

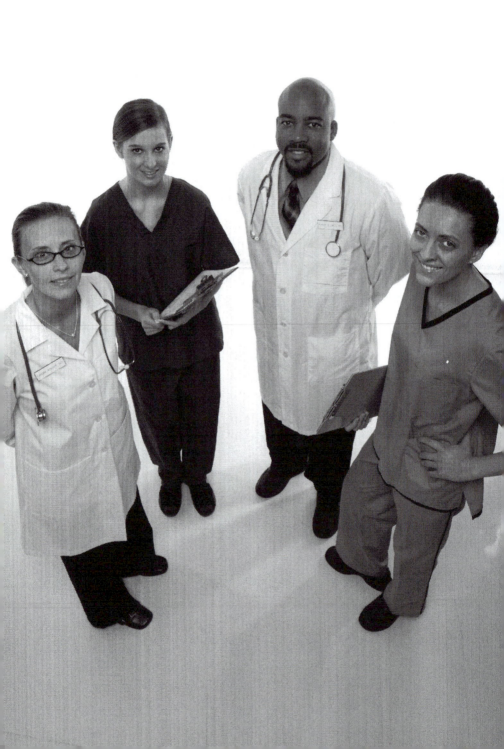

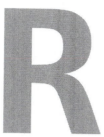

Relationships

A leader takes people where they want to go. A great leader takes people where they don't necessarily want to go but ought to be.

Rosalynn Carter

A s a leader, the relationships you have with your teams, your peers, your own manager, yourself and your friends and family outside the work environment are all crucial to successfully fulfilling your role. Each relationship is different, and each contributes in a different way to your effectiveness as a leader. But perhaps the most important relationship to nurture and nourish is the one that you have with yourself – for this is where that all important confidence, conviction and self-authentic behaviour is derived.

As a clinician working with patients on a day-to-day basis, you will no doubt have frequently received praise for the work that you undertook. Patients say 'thank you' all the time; and their family bring in tokens of their gratitude, sending cards, flowers, confectionery and donations to the staff, ward or unit that looked after their mother, father, daughter or son. Clinicians find that their abilities, purpose and talents are praised and validated by others routinely, and thus it can be very difficult to adjust to an environment where the level of praise received is dimmed.

As you move from being a clinician to becoming a leader, and thus become further removed from daily patient praise and managerial support, the level of validation and encouragement you receive reduces dramatically –

it becomes an expectation that your work is effective, efficient, innovative, resourceful. Successfully fulfilling your role is not something that warrants continual praise and encouragement. This is expected. This is the norm. To continue to fulfil your role without recognition of the work you are undertaking can be deflating, particularly if your clinical background has meant that you've received a significant amount of praise and encouragement in the past. But as a leader, there needs to be an understanding that external validation of your work will be rare. Try to remember this when you liaise with your own manager, or those higher up in the hierarchy. Provide them with a little bit of that all-important feedback and encouragement. They will be just as deprived of praise as you are, if not more so.

So, with ever-decreasing levels of validation and positive feedback in the workplace, where do you turn to for that vital encouragement and support? You must look within and pull some self-validation and confidence out from yourself; learning to be self-reliant takes time but is essential in a leadership role. But you can and should also look towards your friends and family for that external validation that is lost within the workplace; seek their reassurance and feedback, and gain positive reinforcement from their comments and support. Of course, let them know that you need this level of encouragement from them so that they have the opportunity to fulfil your needs in this way.

Becoming a leader requires an adjustment within the relationship you hold with yourself, your superiors, and your friends and family. It also requires a change in peer group, and the relationships you hold with an ever-moving group of peers. Most clinicians tend to stick within their own profession, department, team or specialty, building peer relationships with those closest to them. I'm sure we can all think of a time when we 'defended our own' at the cost of another profession or specialty. In fact, in a study that looked into the values and beliefs held by healthcare clinician and non-clinician managers, a key conclusion was that there is general lack of peer cohesion and a large amount of professional conflict within healthcare, highlighted by examples of 'nurse–physician power bases and conflict between clinicians and non-clinicians which manifested in intra-disciplinary control and conflict'.[71] This conflict between clinical and non-clinician managers often occurs because the two 'types' of individuals approach various issues from very different knowledge and value bases. To reconcile the potential for conflict the positives of varying perspectives should be sought, as opposed to viewing each other as enemies fighting for different outcomes.

As you move from being a clinician to a leader your peer group changes, and so those professional or team identities that you held before, and those intra-disciplinary conflicts that you may have been a part of in the past, have to change. Other clinicians may not now be your peer group – they may well be the team of individuals you are responsible for leading. General management or other clinician leaders may become your peer group, and to become a successful leader there is a need to recognise and respect this new peer group and build sustainable relationships with them.

And then of course there are those relationships you have with your staff. A high-performing team needs to be committed to open communication, with strong personal and professional relationships where 'people feel they can take risks and share thoughts, opinions, and feelings without fear'.[72] How team members treat each other and

---

71 Carney, M. 'Positive and Negative Outcomes from Values and Beliefs Held by Healthcare Clinician and Non-clinician Managers', *Journal of Advanced Nursing*, 2006, Vol. 54, No. 1, p114.

72 Blanchard, K. *Leading at a Higher Level*, FT Prentice Hall, Pearson, Harlow, 2007, p170.

how you, as a leader, treat them, impacts on the entire team's ability to 'get the job done'. 'Healthy relationships take practice, are guided by some basic principles (such as trust, mutual respect, consistent and visual support, and open and honest communication), and require ongoing reinforcement.'[73] In addition, individual team members need to feel empowered, and as their leader your relationship with them should be one that encourages empowered self-direction and open communication. Blanchard[74] states that there are three key drivers to empowerment, and these should be incorporated into your leadership style where possible:

1. Sharing information with everyone.

2. Creating autonomy through boundaries; enabling individuals to see how their role fits into the bigger picture, in terms of their immediate team, service and organisation.

3. Replacing hierarchy with self-directed individuals and teams.

Forging strong relationships with staff is an area where those leaders with a clinical background tend to excel. Carney states that managerial receptiveness is an area through which clinicians adopt a caring and supportive approach, resulting in staff feeling valued for their contributions.[75] Pull on this skill; build strong relationships with your team. Empower your staff, team and organisation.

73 Creative Nursing Management, *Leading an Empowered Organisation*, University of Leeds, Handout, 1994.
74 See note 72, pp74–82.
75 See note 71.

Taking relationships forward

▌ Think about your relationship with your manager or leader. Do you provide them with praise or recognition for their work?

▌ Reflect upon Blanchard's drivers to empowerment. What practical steps can you take to integrate these principles in your leadership style?

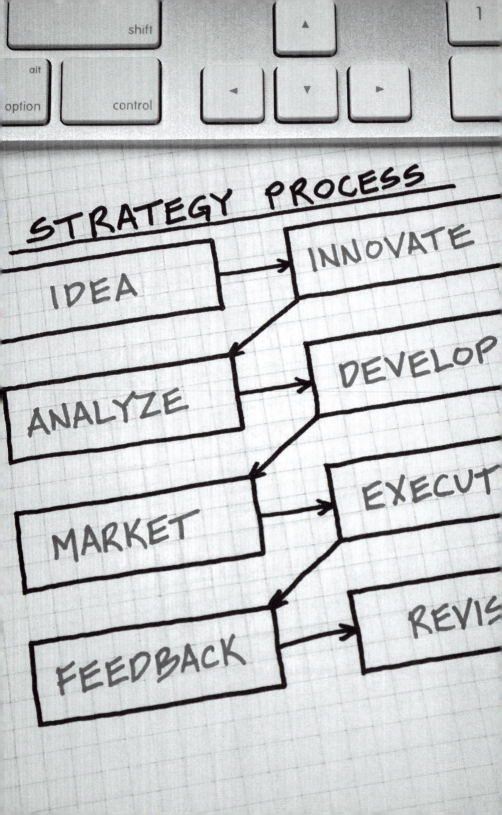

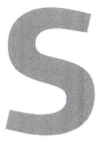

Strategy

Plan your work for today and every day, then work your plan.

Norman Vincent Peale

For any team or organisation to meet the lofty ideals set out in its vision statement it is necessary to have a clear plan and agreed timeframes. This vision is normally the desired or intended future state of the organisation in terms of such things as productivity or turnover. However, within a healthcare situation the desired vision is more likely to relate to areas such as introducing new and improved services, waiting times, infection control standards or patient experience. In order to achieve this vision a clearly defined and structured plan needs to be developed and subsequently implemented. This plan can be defined as the strategy. The vision that is used to set the future standards is very important and in defining it you will decide the success or failure of the strategy. 'A vision must be realistic, attainable, credible, challenging and attractive to those in the organisation.'[76] If the vision is fundamentally unattainable then there is no purpose in composing a strategy to reach it as this will never be accomplished and will not only be detrimental to the organisation but will also reflect poorly on you as a leader. The vision must be right in order that the strategy can be successfully implemented. 'The most important foundation of a health-care organisation's success

76 Barker, A.M., Sullivan, D.T. and Emery, M.J. *Leadership Competencies for Clinical Managers: The Renaissance of Transformational Leadership*, Jones and Bartlett, London, 2005, p106.

is visionary leadership, for the whole organisation, and for each unit or department.'[77] To try to lead without a strategy would be extremely unproductive as without a focus or a plan you will make many errors and work ineffectively on the way to achieving your vision, which without a strategy may indeed never be obtained.

Strategic planning is the process that is used in most organisations to deliver the vision. There is a definite methodology to developing and implementing a strategic plan and there are some suggested steps that should be followed when doing so. These steps are defined as follows:

1. Scan the internal environment.
2. Conduct a scan of the external environment.
3. Conduct a SWOT (strengths, weaknesses, opportunities, threats) analysis.
4. Create or revise the vision, if needed.
5. Develop strategic initiatives.
6. Implement strategic plans.
7. Evaluate the results.[78]

Most leaders know their organisations very well and will generally understand or at least have a good sense of the strategies that are required for success. Therefore working through points 1 to 5 above will not necessarily raise too many challenges. However, the problem lies in the delivery of the strategy. Leaders often fail to put their theory into action so that the well thought out strategy that should be successful actually fails to achieve the vision. In *The Times 1000*, a study of 200 companies showed that 80 per cent of directors believed that they had the right strategies but only 14 per cent thought that they were implementing them well.[79] A good leader therefore will not only be able to create a sound strategic plan but they will also possess the necessary skills to deliver it effectively. There are certain leadership qualities that will facilitate the successful implementation of a strategy. The first of these is motivational leadership. This is an essential element that will help the process of translating strategy into results. Being able to motivate and engage staff in the strategic plan will give them the drive to put the plan into action. To engage staff you should try to involve them in the detail of the strategic plan. A good leader will make their team understand the intent behind the strategy and its aims so that they are aware of the objectives they are working towards and the reasons for doing so. Providing this knowledge will help to ensure that the whole team is working towards a common goal and with a unified approach. Another leadership skill that can be applied to ensure strategy success is that of performance management. Setting individual targets and work plans that are in line with the strategic plan will aid its implementation by ensuring that your team remain focused on the strategy and the underlying vision. There should then follow a systematic way of measuring progress against these targets through regular assessment and feedback, which will help to reaffirm the long-term strategy.

Evaluating the success of a strategy and your progress towards the vision is an essential part of strategic planning. In order to assess whether your strategy process is working you can look at key business results or key performance indicators (KPIs). These will provide a measurable quantitative or qualitative guide by which you can measure progress and your strategy's success. The situation may arise where you conclude that the strategy is not effective and should therefore be redefined. A good leader should be able to recognise this situation and should not hesitate to adjust the strategy accordingly.

The strategic plan is generally long term but it should always be referred to when constructing short-term plans and when analysing progress and providing feedback to your team. Your strategy should be the driving force behind all your leadership decisions and actions. By working in conjunction with the strategy you will ultimately be more productive as a leader and you will eventually achieve the vision.

Taking strategy forward

▌ Using the seven steps outlined at the start of this chapter, evaluate a strategy which you have across your team, department or organisation. How does your strategy look when under close scrutiny?

▌ Reflect upon the ways in which you have implemented a strategy. This could be something as simple as a minor clinical practice change right through to a new initiative. What would you have done better to link strategy and implementation?

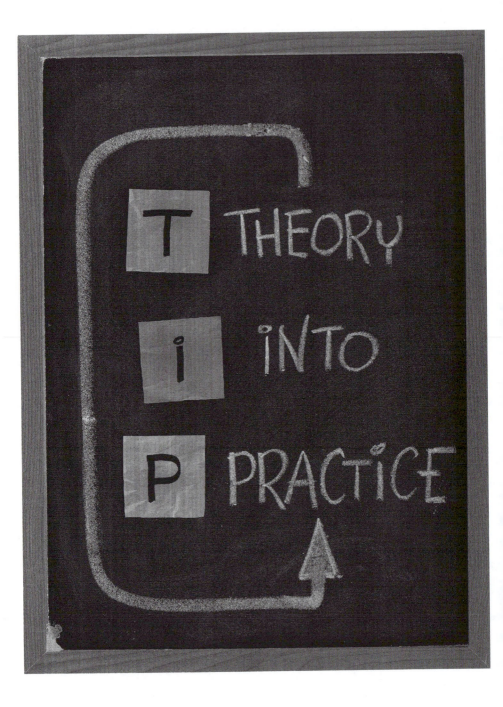

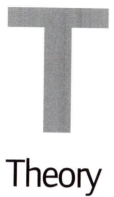

Theory

I start with the premise that the function of leadership is to produce more leaders, not more followers.

Ralph Nader

There are many leadership theories that have emerged over the years, several of which provide a good structure for effective leadership. However, this chapter is not concerned with debating the value or merits of any of these theories, but is simply here to express the importance of using theory in leadership practice.

A 'theory' is a researched idea that has been tested and validated to produce a framework to guide practice. Such evidence-based approaches provide a degree of certainty within your practice as there is proof that this method has previously produced the desired outcome. As a leader, understanding and using theory will enable you to work with confidence around a tried and tested model, and it will also enhance your knowledge and understanding. Many healthcare leaders will come from one of the caring professions. Nursing has probably led the way in developing and using underpinning philosophical theories to enable practitioners to better understand the situations they see before them. Those theories frequently have a humanistic core. However, all clinical disciplines are now well grounded in evidence-based practice – in other words, 'theory'. Leaders, regardless of their professional background, may find it beneficial to read some nursing theory because so much of it can be used in unpicking and understanding the complex and chaotic world of healthcare, the people we serve and the challenges of clinical practice. This is all about moving from evidence-based clinical practice, so familiar to clinicians, to evidence-based leadership practice. The idea that theory improves your knowledge, which in turn enhances your inherent power, implies that theory should always be the driving force behind an effective leader.

Simply being aware of theory is not sufficient in itself: embedding it in practice and keeping up to date is the next challenge. A successful healthcare leader should regularly read journals and articles to make sure that they are fully informed of new approaches and developments in different environments and contexts. Reading on a routine basis will not only increase your knowledge, it will also help you to develop leadership skills. For example, in nursing, 'the study of theory helps develop analytical skills, challenge thinking, clarify values and assumptions, and determine purposes for nursing practice'.[80]

One theorist whose work can very much be applied to leadership practice is Margaret A. Newman. Her work is based around the ideas of consciousness, movement, relationships and time and space. Her concept is actually a nursing theory. However, at the root of it are some fascinating ideas about energy. This might all seem rather esoteric but before dismissing it think about her work and how it might relate to the negative energy in an ineffective team and how that team's performance can be made better. In its original form this theory clearly applies to clinical practice but the concepts around it can also be considered in terms of leadership. As a leader you should not simply be focused on meeting targets, you should instead be guided by the desire to improve your team's effectiveness in order

---

[80] Tomey, M.R. and Alligood, A.M. *Nursing Theorists and Their Work*, 4th edition, Mosby, MO, 1998, p3.

to achieve improved levels of patient care. This approach works along the lines of servant leadership. This second theory is one that many organisations have adopted and should be fundamental to the approach of healthcare leaders. Servant leadership theory, by definition, is the act of leading whilst being driven by the desire to serve. In healthcare terms this equates to an effective leader working with a strong desire to improve patient care and serve patients and the organisation they work within. This desire is the reason why people become clinicians in the first place. A servant leader adapts these core values of clinicians to make a difference as a leader. A servant leader should have 'a natural feeling that one wants to first serve others that leads one to aspire to lead others';[81] they should also have 'a commitment to help others grow as persons'.[82] Working as a servant leader will allow you to remain mindful of your purpose whilst improving your performance and that of your team.

Failing to recognise or ignoring the importance of theory, and particularly the merits of nursing theory as a leadership tool, can be detrimental in several ways. First, this ignorance can lead to a personal detachment from your original objectives in respect to improving healthcare. Neglecting theory may allow for an unfocused leadership role to develop, which distracts from your core values and will hinder your attempts to drive forward agendas. Second, once you lose sight of your goals, the team that you are leading could potentially disengage as they realise that you are no longer authentic, or respecting or following proven methodologies, both clinically and within leadership. In addition, dismissing any theory without fully understanding or analysing it suggests a certain degree of arrogance,

81 Milstead, J.A. and Furlong, E. *Handbook of Nursing Leadership: Creative Skills for a Culture of Safety*, Jones and Bartlett, London, 2006, p7.
82 See note above.

implying that you are completely knowledgeable and do not believe that you can enhance your understanding any further! This, of course, is never the case and a good leader should always be a life-long learner looking to know more, understand more and apply theory in their everyday working life. They should always be aware that 'theory helps provide knowledge to improve practice'.[83]

Taking theory forward

▌ Read Margaret A. Newman's *Health as Expanding Consciousness*.[84]

▌ Read about servant leadership and reflect on why it is energising and enabling.

▌ Identify a piece of evidence-based leadership and consider implementing it.

---

83 Tomey, M.R. and Alligood, A.M. *Nursing Theorists and Their Work*, 4th edition, Mosby, MO, 1998, p3.
84 Newman, M.A. *Health as Expanding Consciousness*, 2nd edition, Jones and Bartlett (NLN Press), Sudbury, MA, 1999.

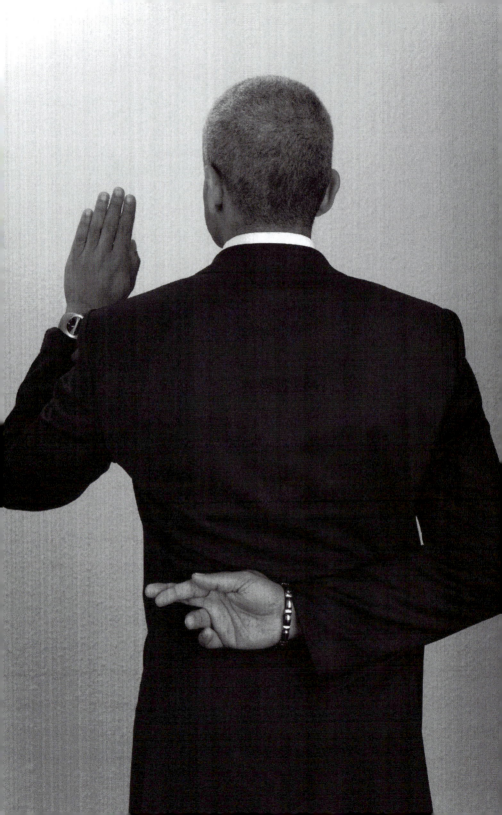

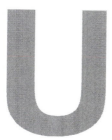

Unethical leadership

Nothing can stop the man with the right mental attitude from achieving his goal; nothing on earth can help the man with the wrong mental attitude.

Thomas Jefferson

Many positive forms of leadership style are discussed throughout this book, and there are copious other leadership books that discuss in great detail various leadership strategies, with differing forms of servant leadership perhaps being one of the most contemporary styles of positive leadership currently recognised. There does, however, need to be some acknowledgement of how *not* to do it. By recognising the common traits of unethical or poor leadership styles, you can ensure that whichever leadership strategy you adopt, you don't choose a style that is detrimental to both yourself and those around you.

Unethical leadership can be classified as leadership that goes against commonly accepted moral standards. These moral standards include concepts such as honesty, equality, fairness, kindness and acting in an honourable way. By default then, unethical behaviour, and therefore unethical leadership, involves behaviour that is false or untrue, fails to respect diversity, is unjust or unfair, mean or unkind and deceitful. This behaviour works against all of the ideals set out in servant leadership, which include authenticity, trustworthiness, self-awareness, an understanding of the values of others, visibility, openness and integrity.

Three principal unethical leadership strategies exist, and strands of each can often be seen in poor leadership styles.

These unethical strategies are co-dependent leadership, coercive leadership and self-serving leadership.

Co-dependent leadership

Co-dependency has been defined as 'a pattern of detrimental behavioural interactions with others'.[85] A leader who is co-dependent relies on the actions, thoughts or views of another to survive. This level of dependence in a leader is unwise for a number for reasons. First, as we have seen in the chapter on Relationships, taking on the role of a leader changes the relationships that you have with other individuals. Those who were once your peers become your staff – people who depend on you to lead them – not the other way round! The higher up the leadership food chain you go, the greater your responsibility to lead a team, service or hospital independently becomes; with interaction and advice from others, yes, but without the need to rely on their encouraging actions or opinions. As a leader you have to learn to become independent, self-reliant and self-confident in your decisions and actions as the level of praise, recognition and encouragement you receive from others drops. This may be quite a change for some clinicians who, since starting in healthcare, will have become used to the loveliness of patients and relatives providing constant positive feedback and sincere thanks. As a leader you'll need to get used to not being thanked, or even being unpopular!

Secondly, the personality traits associated with co-dependency can detrimentally affect how others view, trust and respect you as a leader. The behaviour of a co-dependent leader might include controlling others, distrusting others, expecting unachievable perfection, and

85 Cermark, T. 'Children of Alcoholics and the Case for a New Diagnostic Category of Co-dependency', *Alcohol Health and Research World*, 1984, 8(4), pp38–42.

a difficulty in expressing feelings or viewpoints. Failing to give individuals responsibility or autonomy, distrust and placing undue pressure on a team to produce unattainable results quickly leads to a demotivated, untrusting and unproductive workforce. This is certainly not the sort of group an effective leader is looking to create. An effective team is led by a confident leader who is present, authentic, trusted and motivating. This team cannot be built or led through co-dependency.

Coercive leadership

Coercion goes against key positive leadership skills and concepts such as mentorship, engagement, humanity, relationship building and influence. Coercion involves forcing an individual to do something through intimidation, force or bullying. It can also involve oppressing their personal values or opinions in order to get a particular task completed.

Be careful not to underestimate the negative impact that coercive leadership can have, both on your ability to lead a successful team and on the individuals that you are leading. Being a victim of intimidation or bullying at work can seriously affect the mental and emotional health of an individual, especially if it is their manager or leader who is the pursuing this behaviour. Coercive leadership will almost definitely lead to increased stress levels in staff, which in turn is likely to reduce productivity, reduce efficiency, reduce motivation, increase sickness levels and negatively affect staff retention. However, it is vital for a leader to be clear in their own mind about the difference between bullying and performance management. This is because almost every accomplished leader has faced situations in which their attempts to performance-manage individuals who are failing to meet their job descriptions or objectives have been misconstrued as bullying.

Self-serving leadership

Being self-serving means ensuring that all of your actions benefit yourself first and foremost. There is a wonderful Northern saying that sums up this concept wonderfully. It is, 'If thee ever does owt for nowt, always do it for thee sen', which roughly translates as, 'If you ever do anything for free, always make sure it benefits you'. Whereas servant leadership is born out of a desire to act in a way which benefits others, self-serving leadership comes through a desire to always benefit and promote yourself. In any organisation a leader whose primary focus is their own well-being will quickly find they lose the respect, trust and support of others. In healthcare, where you are surrounded by individuals who strive to care for others on a daily basis, there is really no place for self-serving attitudes as they are diametrically opposed to the values of servant leadership to which many clinicians relate. According to Miller and Ross, self-serving leadership occurs when 'leaders attribute their successes to personal factors but attribute their failures to factors beyond their control. Self-serving leadership can be seen as the human tendency to take credit for success but to deny the responsibility for failure.'[86] A key leadership behavioural principle is that of self-awareness, particularly in relation to 'failures'. Failures are learning opportunities and it's really important to use such opportunities to reflect and improve one's leadership practice.

Avoiding unethical leadership

▌ Develop a thorough understanding of your organisation's harassment and bullying policy, and their policy on managing poor performance. Can you use these appropriately and ethically?

86 Miller, D.T. and Ross, M. 'Self-serving Biases in the Attribution of Causality: Fact or Fiction?', *Psychological Bulletin*, 1975, 82, pp213–225.

▌ Reflect upon an example of unethical leadership that you have observed. How can you best guard against such a style of leadership in your own practice or amongst people you work with?

▌ Research and reflect upon the Nolan Committee's 'Seven Principles of Public Life', which are Selflessness, Integrity, Objectivity, Accountability, Openness, Honesty and Leadership. Evaluate the impact of these on you as a leader.

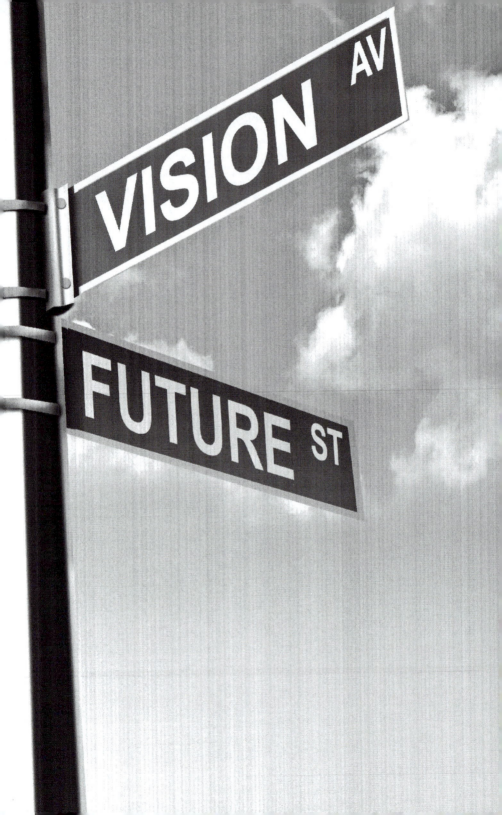

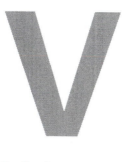

Vision

Never doubt that a small group of thoughtful,
concerned citizens can change the world. Indeed it is
the only thing that ever has.

Margaret Mead

Vision is vital in order to be able to plan strategies and to motivate and lead others towards a defined goal. All good leaders should ensure that they have a clear vision of where they want themselves, their team and their organisation to be in the future. Visionary leadership 'paints an inspiring picture of what an organisation can become'.[87]

One of the key traits of an effective leader is having the ability to provide vision for the future, which in turn provides others with confidence and inspiration to follow their lead. Once a vision has been conceived, a good leader should then be able to define a direction that everyone within their organisation can share with them and follow in order to achieve that vision. This direction can be formally worked into strategic plans, which will reaffirm the organisation's goal and describe how the processes and steps they plan to put in place will achieve that vision. In order for the vision to actually be realised and for people to actively follow your lead and to have the same focus in their work, it is essential that you establish the right environment for your staff. This environment should allow them the opportunity to grow and develop so that they are not limited by their resources on the way to achieving the vision. It is also important to note that for a vision to be used effectively to inspire and motivate others, it is essential that it is solid, and not one that consists of weak statements or unrealistic concepts.

As well as providing a focus for people's work, a vision also dramatises new directions that others might not buy into otherwise. As such, a vision is a useful tool for facilitating change. A clear vision is invaluable for those who may be resistant to change and need something clear and concise to focus on in order to picture the desired goal.

One of the best ways to define your vision and to inform others of it is to create a vision statement that defines and communicates the organisation's purpose and values. This statement should be clear and direct and should act as a contract between the organisation and the patients to inform them about what they should expect. The statement should also provide staff with a focus on how they are expected to behave, and it should inspire and motivate them to give their best in order that they are always working towards the vision. To be able to communicate the vision of an organisation effectively the leader must remember that the vision should not be confused with the mission. Vision is the long-term aim of the organisation, whereas the mission is a higher purpose that focuses on the broader impact the organisation has on society.

There are some fundamental points to remember when developing a vision that is both useful and excites and motivates people to follow a leader. 'The vision must:

▌ clearly set organisational direction and purpose;

▌ inspire loyalty and caring through the involvement of all employees;

▌ display and reflect the unique strengths, culture, values, beliefs and direction of the organisation;

▌ inspire enthusiasm, belief, commitment and excitement in company members;

▌ help employees believe that they are part of something bigger than themselves and their daily work;

▌ be regularly communicated and shared;

▌ challenge people to outdo themselves, to stretch and reach.'[88]

This last point is particularly important as a vision must be something that is aspired to and that can be achieved through improvement and excellence in all areas of the organisation. A vision is pointless if it is easily attainable now without any progress or development needing to be made.

To lead with vision is very important and it should be evident in the actions, beliefs, values and goals of a good leader. If a leader is not able to see a vision and to articulate that vision to others then it can becoming demoralising for those they are leading. If you do not have a clear vision or you are unable to articulate it to your team or, indeed, you do not refer to or adhere to it within your work, then you will not achieve respect as a leader and it is likely that your staff will not be fulfilling their potential. Staff will generally take a lead from your example, therefore if you have made them aware of a clear vision and the steps needed to achieve it, and if you are then seen to be consistently incorporating that vision within your work, your team should be motivated to adopt a similar work ethic so that you are all working together towards the same goal.

Taking vision forward

▌ Using the criteria in this chapter, review your organisation's vision statement. How does it measure up to the criteria? Do you think it helps to guide your work as a leader? If not, consider making some suggestions for changes. If your organisation doesn't have a vision statement consider writing one, either as an exercise in vision statement writing for your own use, or as a suggestion for wider use.

▌ Thinking completely 'out of the box', consider your career vision as a leader. What do you want to achieve? What is important to you? You may want to write down three to four career vision statements.

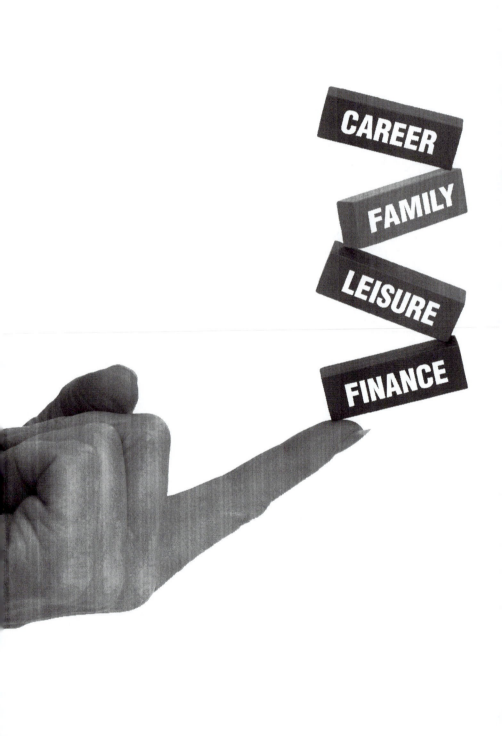

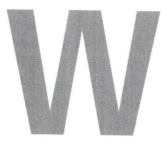

Work–life balance

Our lives are a mixture of different roles. Most of us are doing the best we can to find whatever the right balance is ... For me, that balance is family, work and service.

Hillary Clinton

The case for adopting a good work–life balance is now widely acknowledged across all industries. Some of the many benefits to the organisation are a reduction in sickness absences and other incidents of absenteeism, improved recruitment and retention and a more contented and productive workforce. Benefits to the individual include feeling fulfilled within a range of aspects of their life, such as family and fitness, which in turn gives them more energy and motivation within the workplace. 'Work–life balance is achieved when an individual's right to a fulfilled life inside and outside paid work is accepted and respected as the norm, to the mutual benefit of the individual, business and society.'[89]

Work–life balance was at one time considered only to be of relevance to parents of young children but nowadays everyone appreciates the value of getting the balance right and more and more individuals are adopting the attitude of 'work to live' not 'live to work'. There are many aspects that need to be considered within work–life balance, including holidays, stress management, spiritual nourishment and fulfilling hobbies and interests such as art, music and reading. Individuals today expect flexibility within their work and expect to be able to lead a full family and domestic life whilst also being able to enjoy more individual pastimes and hobbies. An organisation that can provide this type of working environment will not only appear more attractive but also will continue to employ a more effective staff. 'The smartest and most forward-looking organisations will see that by putting work–life balance at the heart of their cultures and their strategic plans they will not only be satisfying employees and creating more equitable workplaces, but increasing their productivity and responding competitively to significant changes, such as our growing 24/7 lifestyle.'[90] There are ways in which you can accommodate staff to ensure that they have the time and freedom to create a good work–life balance. In healthcare, safe patient care is and always must be the top priority. Sometimes this conflicts with individuals' desires because they must work unusual hours, but it is vital that the leader always promotes the priority of patient care.

In the context of leading a clinical service the ideal of flexibility has to be further balanced against patient safety priorities. It simply may not be possible to agree flexible work plans for every clinical member of staff, especially those working in teams where proper continuity requires people to work together at set times each day, for example. It is also important to consider some of the research that indicates that certain shift patterns, such as 12-hour shifts, create a clinical risk.

As a leader you should acknowledge the need for a good work–life balance within your own life and within the lives of your staff. You should endeavour to schedule dedicated time to alternative activities outside the workplace – whether this be a regular sporting activity, participating in amateur dramatics or just spending time reading a book – that isn't

90 Jones, A. *About Time for Change*, The Work Foundation, London, 2003.

work-related! All of these activities will allow you to relax and refocus, which is essential to be a more effective leader, particularly if you work in a high-pressure environment. Establishing a work–life balance is a discipline and there is no 'one size fits all' rule. Every individual will require a different amount of time to be allocated to each aspect of their life and within this, the best allocation of work–life balance could vary over time and from day to day. Thus, as a leader, you should be aware of the need for flexibility within your schedule. For example, at the start of the week you may find that the greatest fulfilment you will experience will come from working a full day and overtime to ensure that a task is completed, but as the week progresses your desires may shift so that you will experience the greatest fulfilment by spending more time with your family or by going to the theatre. You should possess the self-awareness to be able to assess your current state of fulfilment and to act in such a way that you are optimising your work–life balance as much as possible. To obtain a good balance you have to be able to 'switch off' from your work. One theoretically easy way to do this is to physically switch off your work mobile phone or BlackBerry so that you are not tempted to check emails or make telephone calls that could wait until the next working day. In practice this task is actually a very hard thing to do for most leaders, particularly those who are dedicated to their job and feel that they should always be thinking about work.

For committed leaders it is sometimes hard to see the benefits of a good work–life balance as some still believe that to be a workaholic is the only way to succeed within an organisation. However, this is not true and to adopt such a work style is actually quite destructive and ineffective. Therefore as a leader, you should lead by example. Staff who regularly observe leaders starting work early and finishing late can actually start to feel guilty that they themselves are not showing the same level of commitment. As a leader you should be conscious of the impact that your work–life balance has on those that you are leading. By establishing the right combination within your life you will be seen to be more effective at work and will generally demonstrate that you are in a fulfilled and happy state of being. In order to determine the combination that works for you, you should take time to assess your lifestyle and your priorities. When discussing work–life balance a commonly cited theme when prioritising the aspects of your life is to try to both achieve *and* enjoy something each day, in each field of your life such as work, family, etc. 'The "career" challenge for successful leaders demands the creation of a range of priorities and goals which can be enjoyed as opposed to simply achieved.'[91] Once you have determined your priorities and made real efforts to get a balance that works for you, then the benefits to both yourself and to your organisation will soon be evident. If your team can see you showing the positive effects of a good work–life balance then, with your encouragement, they will also understand the need to adopt a similar ethic within their own lives.

Taking work–life balance forward

▮ Take a brutal look at your week. What is the balance between life and work? If in doubt, keep a chart of your activities.

▮ Reflect upon what you've done today to achieve your work goals. Was this an effective use of your time?

▮ Reflect upon what you've done today 'to make you feel good' or, in other words, what have you done for yourself?

91 Clayton, D. *Leadershift – The Work-Life Balance Program*, Acer Press, Camberwell, Vic., 2004, p146.

▌ Look at your timetable for a month. Is your work–life balance in sync with your work–life goals? If not, how will you address this?

▌ Think about what you could do as a leader to improve the work–life balance of the people in your team.

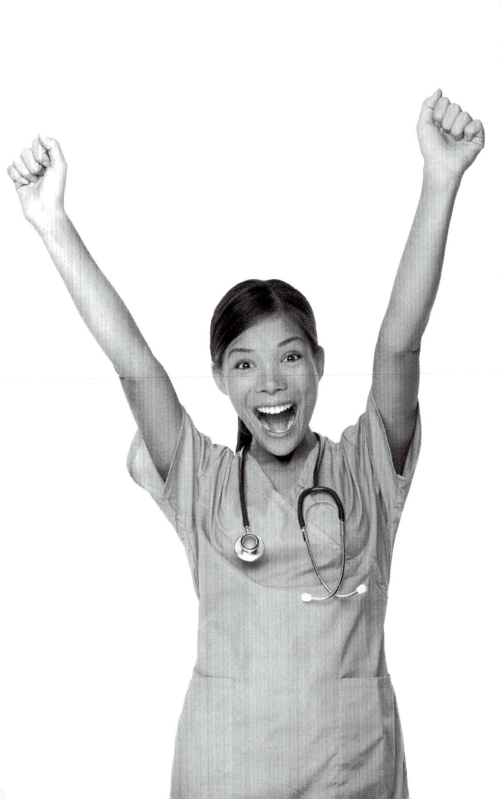

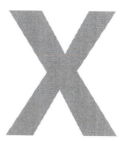

eXcitement

Leaders who can stay optimistic and upbeat, even under intense pressure, radiate the positive feelings that create resonance. By staying in control of their feelings and impulses, they craft an environment of trust, comforts and fairness. And that self-management has a trickle down effect from the leader.

Daniel Goleman

One important concept that leaders should try to promote within their workforce is excitement. Without excitement the workplace can appear dull and uninteresting and will not be an environment in which staff will feel motivated to give their best. A good leader will try to keep the workplace alive with excitement, thus making it somewhere that people look forward to coming to, and somewhere that will sustain their interest in their work. As a leader you should also be enthusiastic about work and delivering your best. This enthusiasm and commitment will then rub off on others and have a knock-on effect on your team which encourages them to show the same level of commitment. To be excited you also need to possess a certain amount of energy, although not too much, as individuals portraying excessive energy can be considered to be unauthentic and could be thought of as insincere in their approach. A moderate amount of energy therefore, joined with an upbeat, positive attitude, will encourage others to feel the same way and to be excited about their work. The presence of excitement, positivity and energy will result in a much happier work ethos and well-motivated staff.

Excitement is also a vital concept within change management. Healthcare is constantly evolving and as such new processes and schools of thought about the best ways of working are inevitably being implemented. These will nearly always involve change, which may unnerve some of the team. If as a leader you approach change with a positive and 'can do' attitude then this will influence others and encourage them to adopt a similar stance. A feeling of excitement about change rather than dread will create a better working ethos and will help you to lead the change.

There are ways to encourage excitement; the first is to ensure you have a complementary mix of staff within your team. A ward or clinical environment is just like any other situation where many people must work together in order to achieve similar goals.[92] Some of these individuals will be extroverted and very outgoing in their nature, whilst others will be more introverted and more likely not to speak up, going along with the majority opinion to keep the peace. Those that are extrovert can often make the office an exciting place, and create a fun atmosphere in which to work. Some will find this very motivating and uplifting whilst the more introvert may find this attitude to be overpowering and quite daunting. This may have a negative impact on their work and behaviour and lead to underperformance. So getting the balance right is vital. Within your staff mix there will be many differing personalities and each of these will require different things to inspire them. It is important then to get to know your workforce so that you are able to determine what makes them tick and therefore how to get them to be excited about their day-to-day work.

The next step to deliver excitement within your team is to ensure that your employees are excited by their workloads. This is not a constantly viable situation, and no leader should expect to be able to continuously deliver this. One way of initiating excitement is by allowing employees to change their normal work pattern or to lead on different

92 www.essortment.com/different-personalities-36352.html

areas. Not only will this bring excitement for the employee but also for you as a leader, as you will be able to see your team gain confidence, expand and develop. Staff development can also be achieved by allowing personnel to attend training courses that will expand their knowledge and understanding, and will consequently be of benefit to both the employee, the team and the organisation. Keeping up to date with changes that affect their daily routine will keep the employee motivated and will also make them feel more involved in their role. Allowing staff to progress and develop in this way will hopefully instill some excitement and positivity. Other things that can also be done in the workplace to make it more challenging and to bring something a little different to the usual working day include holding simple events like a staff lunch, or a team away day. These types of morale-boosting occasions help in bringing a team together and add some excitement. Another example is to initiate a new way to deliver a normally mundane piece of work, which can also have positive effects on staff and create a feeling of excitement for all.

The key to providing an exciting place to work and a feeling of excitement within your team is to lead by example. As a leader you should feel excited about your role and the impact that your efforts will have on the organisation and on patient care. You should be motivated, enthused and excited by your work and should be able to express this, either directly or indirectly. If you appear to be excited and enthused by your role and importance within the organisation it is likely that others will follow suit. An excited team will be a motivated, productive and effective group who will develop and achieve success in line with the organisation's values and the goals and vision set by you as a leader.

Taking excitement forward

▌ Think about how you approach your role. Do you operate with sufficient energy and emotional expression to enthuse those around you?

▌ Remember the importance of balance! A leader who is too excited may have a tendency to cause stress within a team or organisation. On the other hand, a leader who is too restrained can struggle to motivate. It's all about balance! Brainstorm how you can get this balance right in your day-to-day duties.

▌ What changes can you make to your team's role responsibilities to surprise and delight?

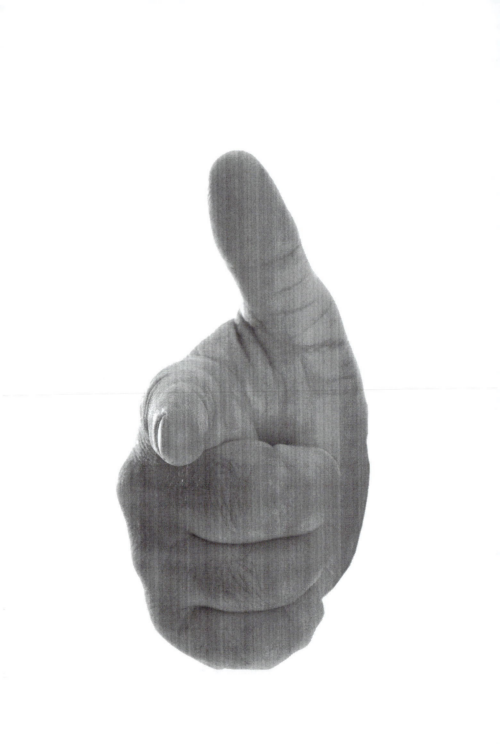

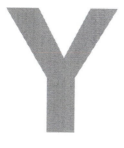

You

The first and best victory is to conquer self.

Plato

According to the *Harvard Business Review*, 'Leadership's First Rule is to – Know Thyself.'[93] Indeed, in order to understand how to be an effective leader it is essential to understand yourself and appreciate your own skills, natural behaviours and skills gaps. To be aware of yourself as a whole person will enable you to make judgements and decisions as to how you can best utilise your qualities and change behaviours to make yourself the most effective leader that you can be.

You must therefore be able to reflect upon and understand what makes you, you. In essence, you must become very self-aware. Aware of how others perceive you, aware of the behaviours that work for you as a leader and aware of those behaviours that need improvement. To be self-analytical and possibly self-critical in such a way can be difficult, first because it is hard to stand back and take an objective view of yourself and second because it is hard to accept that you may have skills gaps that need addressing. Good leaders are normally aware of their strengths and weaknesses. Typically they also have a sense of humour! They normally welcome and accept criticism and feedback that is constructive for their work and therefore facilitates their understanding of themselves, which enables them to develop as a leader. Emotions and self-awareness are inherently linked. Leaders who are emotionally self-aware are more authentic, are more in tune with their emotions and can speak more openly and honestly to those around them. This may enable them to be regarded with greater respect than a leader who is guarded and emotionally unaware. Increasing your levels of self-awareness will allow you to make better decisions, get more out of your colleagues, communicate more effectively, and may even help to reduce your own stress levels.

Once you have established a greater sense of self-awareness and understanding of your emotions and behaviours, the next step is self-management. Having determined the behaviours that need to change you then have to manage the change. In order to achieve this you will need to reflect on your actions and interactions with others. A degree of perseverance is required in order that you can make these changes a permanent feature of your leadership style. Self-management also relates to the need to manage your emotions and your inner self to allow for the focus that all leaders need in order to achieve their vision and their goals. Managing emotion effectively is vital. The emotions that a leader is feeling are often passed on to their staff, therefore it is important that the feelings that your colleagues pick up on are ones of a positive nature so that they too can emulate them. Leaders who are able to stay in control of their emotions and present themselves in a professional, calm and collected manner are more likely to be seen as more effective leaders by their staff. To be able to self-manage your emotions also allows you a greater understanding of feelings generally, which will help you to better deal with the emotions of those around you. 'Leaders cannot effectively manage emotions in anyone else without first handling their own.'[94] Being able to 'assess and manage the emotions of oneself,

---

[94] Goleman, D., Boyatzis, R. and McKee, A. *The New Leaders: Transforming the Art of Leadership into the Science of Results,* Little Brown, London, 2002, p46.

of others'[95] is to possess a degree of emotional intelligence. This emotional intelligence is an essential quality for an effective leader as it allows them to connect with their team in order that they can draw the best from them. A high level of emotional intelligence may be considered by some as a more desirable quality to be demonstrated by a leader than a high IQ.

In addition to self-awareness, self-management and emotional intelligence, an effective leader also needs to possess a certain sense of self-belief. 'Self confidence is the fundamental basis from which leadership grows.'[96] Without self-confidence leadership cannot exist effectively. A good leader must have the confidence to make important decisions that affect their team and their patients. A good leader must believe in their goals and their values and have the confidence to stand by their beliefs and ideals. Without self-confidence you will not convince others that the decisions you have made or the actions that you are implementing are the right ones. If you do not believe in yourself and your work then others will be inclined to follow your lead and not believe in you either.

Self-confidence is a quality that develops over time and grows as you prove yourself as a competent leader. To be and to appear to be a competent leader requires a great deal of inward-looking analysis. You will have to assess and reassess your leadership skills, your values and your behaviours time and time again to ensure that you are delivering your best. You must understand yourself and act upon the things that you find out about your personality to allow yourself to change and improve. 'A sense of self is not about selfishness, or self-absorption. The objective isn't to be yourself, the challenge is to be your best self.'[97]

95 Bradberry, T. and Greaves, J. *Emotional Intelligence 2.0*, Group West, San Francisco, 2009.

96 www.inc.com/resources/leadership

97 www.marksanborn.com

Taking you forward

▌ Reflect on 'you' as a leader. Write down three of your best leadership qualities and three skills that require development. Create a plan to celebrate your best leadership qualities (even if it's just applauding yourself or buying yourself a present!) and make a plan for improving your skills in your three areas for development.

▌ Reflect upon a situation in which you have positively used 'you' to improve the care of a group of patients or an individual patient. What did you do well? What could you improve upon next time you are faced with something similar?

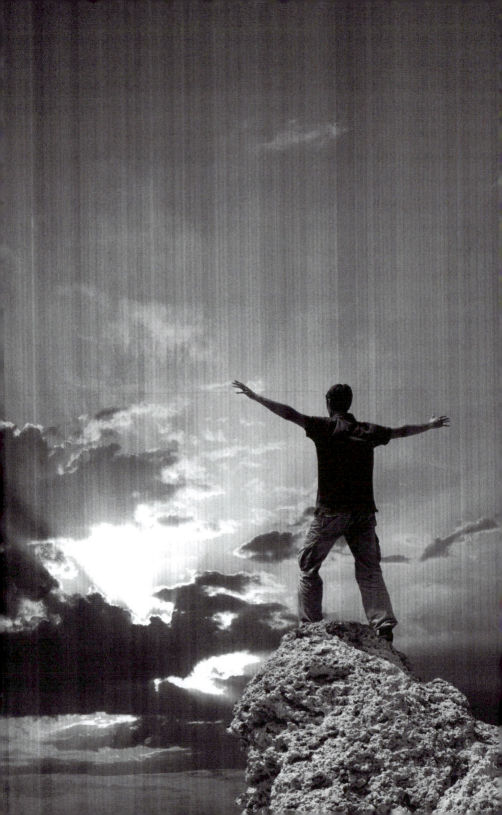

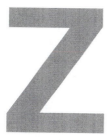

Zenith

*Celebrate what you've accomplished, but raise the bar
a little higher each time you succeed.*

Mia Hamm

The term 'zenith' is defined by the Oxford Dictionary as the time at which something is most powerful or successful.[98] In contemporary language the word zenith isn't widely used any more, but for the purposes of this chapter we will use the term as a definition for recognising the peak of one's career, and discuss the importance of celebrating a peak or overall achievement. The achievements or successes that you as a leader should celebrate can be both personal and career-focused, and can be your own individual achievements, or those of your team and indeed wider organisation.

As acknowledged in previous chapters, as you move further and further up the hierarchical food chain, the internal recognition of your achievements begins to dwindle. Whilst in previous roles patients, peers and management may have thanked you for your hard work and dedication, or may have celebrated a significant achievement, as leaders most people find that their successes and achievements become expected as opposed to celebrated. Without celebration or recognition of your successes it can be very difficult to retain motivation and enthusiasm for your job, role or career path. And so, as a leader, it is important that you take time to recognise and celebrate your own achievements. These could be milestones that you have reached within your career, or those outside work such as sporting or academic successes.

A proactive and ongoing means of recognising your own achievements is to ensure you always have an up-to-date CV. Take the time to update it frequently, and focus on your achievements within your career. Your CV should show four to five key achievements that you have attained in each role you have held, and these could range from leading a project successfully, turning around the motivation and aptitude of a team, or positively mentoring an individual. These achievements should be related to peak performances within your career roles, and should help to focus your mind on celebrating your personal successes as a leader.

Celebrating your own achievements helps instill a leadership style that focuses on positive praise and recognition of success in others. The acknowledgement of others' achievements, no matter how small, is extremely motivational both for you as a leader and, importantly, for the individual in question. As explored earlier in the Engagement chapter, continued recognition of achievement, praise and positive constructive feedback enables a culture of positivity, energy, passion and commitment to grow within a team.

The active celebration of a team's achievement as a whole is equally as important as the recognition of individual success and, as the leader of a given team, you should also take time to enjoy and celebrate your achievement within the team's success. It may be, for example, that the team you lead has reached set targets for the month, or made significant operational improvements in a particular patient pathway. The celebration of this development or success can be realised in many different ways, such as team away days, lunch or an evening meal, or by simply buying coffee and cake for the team, directorate or area.

Celebrations of an organisation as a whole, or a specific success where the organisation at large is publicly recognised for its attainment are also important, and as an influential leader within this workplace you too should personally enjoy and partake in these events. Often an organisation will recognise the significant successes of individuals and teams within it, and this recognition can be achieved in many different ways; common examples are bonuses or other incentives for employees. It is also common for organisations to offer schemes and programmes that celebrate the organisation's success.

Two global examples of this level of celebration and recognition of achievement are The Prince's Trust and the National Health Service (NHS) in the UK. The Prince's Trust has 'Celebrate Success' recognition awards.[99] The categories within the programme are Volunteer of the Year, Inspiring Leaders Award and The Prince's Trust Staff Award. The mere existence of these awards demonstrates that The Prince's Trust values their staff and recognises their hard work and achievements on an individual, team and organisational level. Similarly, the NHS often publicly celebrate the successes of their staff. In 2007 they ran 'Celebrating Success in Your NHS'. In this programme staff were honoured for their hard work and achievements within the NHS. Milton Keynes General Hospital, for example, won the award for 'Improved patient access – the right care for patients in the right place'. Their success was built on the implementation of a new project, 'Straight to the Test', for cancer patients. The introduction of this pathway met the challenge of achieving extensive cancer targets and reduced patient access and assessment times.

99 www.princes-trust.org.uk

Taking zenith forward

▌ Set aside some time to reinvigorate your CV and ensure that your Key Achievements are highlighted for each of your recent roles. These should come at the beginning of your CV as they are much more important than your qualifications. 'The proof of the pudding is in the eating'! Once rewritten, make sure that your CV is a live document and is regularly updated.

▌ Take time to celebrate your achievements, even if it's just going out for a pizza with friends and family to celebrate something you have managed to deliver as a leader.

▌ Either take charge of entering your team or organisation into a national competition to recognise your collective achievements or encourage your team to enter themselves.

▌ If it's not in place already, encourage your organisation to develop an internal achievement awards process. A good starting point would be to investigate ways in which other organisations have implemented such awards.

Further reading

Barker, A.M., Sullivan, D.T. and Emery, M.J. (2005) *Leadership Competencies for Clinical Managers: The Renaissance of Transformational Leadership*, Jones and Bartlett, London

Blanchard, K. (2007) *Leading at a Higher Level*, FT Prentice Hall, Pearson, Harlow

Browne, M.N. and Keeley, S.M. (2009) *Asking the Right Questions: A Guide to Critical Thinking*, 9th edition, Pearson, Harlow

Freshwater, D., Taylor, J. and Sherwood, G. (2008) *International Textbook on Reflective Practice in Nursing*, Wiley-Blackwell, Oxford

Gardner, H. (1997) *Leading Minds: An Anatomy of Leadership*, HarperCollins, London

Goleman, D., Boyatzis, R. and McKee, A. (2002) *The New Leaders: Transforming the Art of Leadership into the Science of Results*, Little Brown, London

Goleman, D., Boyatzis, R. and McKee, A. (2002) *Primal Leadership: Realizing the Power of Emotional Intelligence*, Harvard Business School Publishing, Boston, MA

Goodwin, N. (2006) *Leadership in Health Care: A European Perspective*, Routledge Health Management Series, Routledge, London and New York

Greenleaf, R.F. (2002) *Servant Leadership: A Journey into the Nature of Legitimate Power and Greatness*, Paulist Press, New York

Halpern, B.L. and Lubar, K. (2006) *Leadership Presence*, Gotham Books, New York

Irvine, D. and Reger, J. (2006) *The Authentic Leader*, DC Press, Sanford, FL

Lanara, V.A. (1996) *Heroism as a Nursing Value: A Philosophical Perspective*, G. Papanikolaou S.A. Graphic Arts, Athens

MacGregor, Burns, J. (2004) *Transforming Leadership*, Atlantic Monthly Press, New York

Mackoff, B. and Wenet, G. (2001) *The Inner Work of Leaders: Leadership as a Habit of Mind*, Amacom Books, New York

Newman, M.A. (1999) *Health as Expanding Consciousness*, Jones and Bartlett (NLN Press), Sudbury, MA

Northouse, P. (2007) *Leadership: Theory and Practice*, Sage, London

Rogers, E.M. (2003) *Diffusion of Innovations*, 4th edition, Free Press, New York

Senge, P., Scharmer, C., Jaworski, J. and Flowers, B. (2005) *Presence: Exploring Profound Change in People, Organizations and Society*, Nicholas Brealey Publishing, London

Sullivan, E.J. and Garland, G. (2010) *Practical Leadership and Management in Nursing*, Pearson, Harlow

Swindall, C. (2007) *Engaged Leadership: Building a Culture to Overcome Employee Disengagement*, John Wiley & Sons, New Jersey

Wagner, R. and Harter, J. (2006) *The Elements of Great Managing*, Gallup Press, New York

Waldock, T. and Kelly-Rawat, S. (2004) *The 18 challenges of Leadership: A Practical, Structured Way to Develop Your Leadership Talent*, Pearson, Harlow

Wheatley, M.J. (1999) *Leadership and the New Science: Discovering Order in a Chaotic World*, 2nd edition, Berrett-Koehler, San Francisco

Woodroffe, S. (2000) *The Book of Yo!* Capstone, Mankato

Nursing & Health Survival Guides

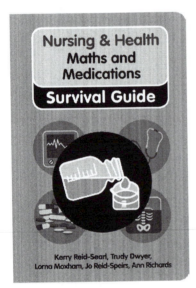

Nursing & Health Maths and Medications
Survival Guide

Kerry Reid-Searl, Trudy Dwyer,
Lorna Moxham, Jo Reid-Speirs, Ann Richards

9780273720225

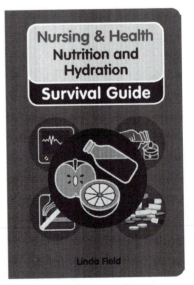

Nursing & Health Nutrition and Hydration
Survival Guide

Linda Field

9780273728719

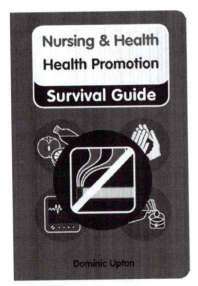

Nursing & Health Health Promotion
Survival Guide

Dominic Upton

9780273728689

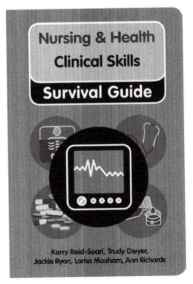

Nursing & Health Clinical Skills
Survival Guide

Kerry Reid-Searl, Trudy Dwyer,
Jackie Ryan, Lorna Moxham, Ann Richards

9780273720478

'A must have for every panicky student!'

Marie-Claire Ratcliffe, Nursing Student

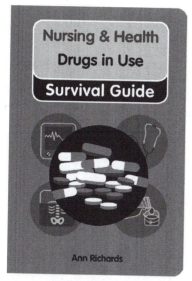

9780273720218

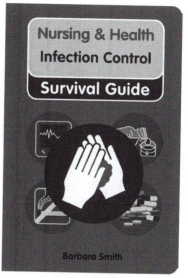

9780273728696

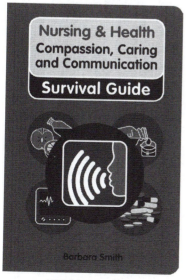

9780273728672

Promoting Healthy Behaviour

A Practical Guide for Nursing and Healthcare Professionals

Dominic Upton & Katie Thirlaway

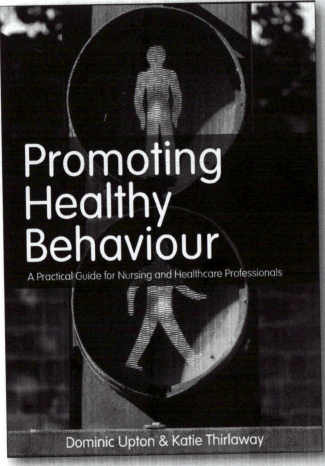

ISBN-13: 9780273723851

'As a nursing student this book has proved invaluable in understanding the theory of health promotion, whilst providing practical ways in which both nurses and other healthcare professionals can apply this theory in practice.'

Natalie Liddle, nursing student, Lincoln University